this is how **ESSENTIAL OILS**

Say Hello

Do you remember the first time you tried Young Living's 100% therapeutic-grade essential oils? It was a profound experience.

We've designed the "Say Hello" series to convey that feeling so that you can share the joy of these remarkable, life-changing products. It's the gift that forever gives...

The Say Hello share kit and tools only from Life Science

1.800.336.6308
www.discoverlsp.com

LIFE SCIENCE™
PRODUCTS & PUBLISHING

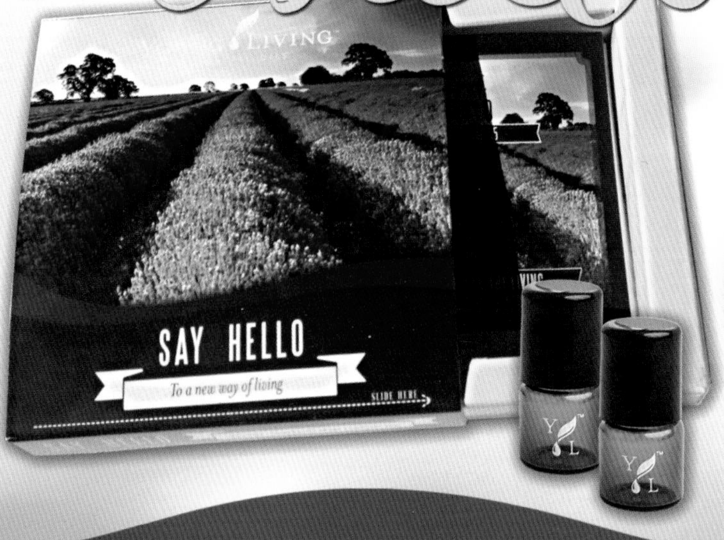

FOREWARD

Congratulations! You've just taken your first step in living a cleaner, greener, more conscientious life. Essential oils are a godsend. They have the power to change people's lives. I happen to know firsthand!

At the age of 21, I was told that I would not live to see 30 because of a serious autoimmune disease. My only chance at survival? Over 15 months of grueling, heartbreaking chemotherapy. It was a long-hard battle—one that I still face every day. And, I couldn't do it without my Young Living Essential Oils.

I'm a long way past 30 (or maybe I've just turned 29 a few times), but I have to say this new lease on life inspired me to make a difference. The past two decades I've devoted myself to the cause of education. But I'm not talking about the make-you- snore-take- a-test- and-forget kind of learning. (Obviously, that has its place. I think...) I'm talking about real knowledge that people can use right away. I'm talking about the self-empowering kind of education, the kind that really frees you to take your life, your health, and your future into your own hands.

In fact, this volume and its many companion volumes are the perfect way to get not only acquainted with essential oils and their many uses, but to do something with them right away. Today, in fact. Every year, my team and I search for the best, most updated information and scientific studies to continue building practical education tools for people to use. It has become an ongoing labor of love and a personal passion. I firmly believe that education is the key to improving the health and lives of everyone in this world.

My company, Life Science Publishing, has been around since Young Living's beginning. While I wasn't there when the doors opened, I certainly know the daily struggles that come with being an entrepreneur. There are constant ups and downs. I can't say they are easy, but I would say they are worth it. I have turned to great mentors in my life, and I believe we can all learn from someone who has been in our shoes before.

Now, I'm not here to sell you oils. I'm here to invite you to learn how they can make a difference in your life—and the lives of the loved ones around you. I'm here to help you get introduced to oils and help you learn how to use them. I would love to say we've met, but if all you know of me is the picture in this book, I hope to meet you soon! I've been told that my energy and passion are contagious. If that's the case, I hope you catch them both...

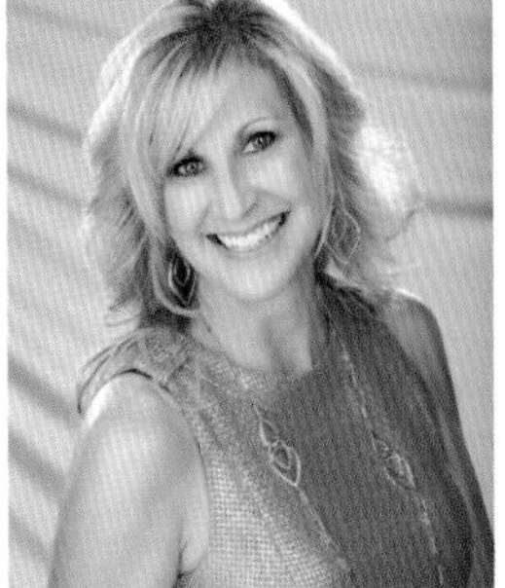

Love. Learn. Share.

xoxo

Troie Battles

Troie Storms-Battles

SAY HELLO TO ESSENTIAL OILS

It's a marvelous world out there—full of the best solutions Mother Nature provides. We want to congratulate you on taking your first steps in living a fuller, richer, healthier life with essential oils. But it goes beyond seeing. The beauty of essential oils is that they go far beyond skin-deep. The benefits of 100% therapeutic grade essential oils can range from the everyday ability to clean sticky tar off a countertop to flavoring the frosting on your gourmet cupcake. They even can bring you closer to the divine.

While these may not seem like miraculous uses, they are profound because essential oils help you to do these things NATURALLY, without petrochemicals, synthetics, coal tar derivatives, petroleum distillates, or laboratory chemicals. In other words, you have the opportunity to be free—free of the forced options of the powerful chemical giants, free from the GMO conglomerates, and even free of the monopolistic pharmaceutical companies.

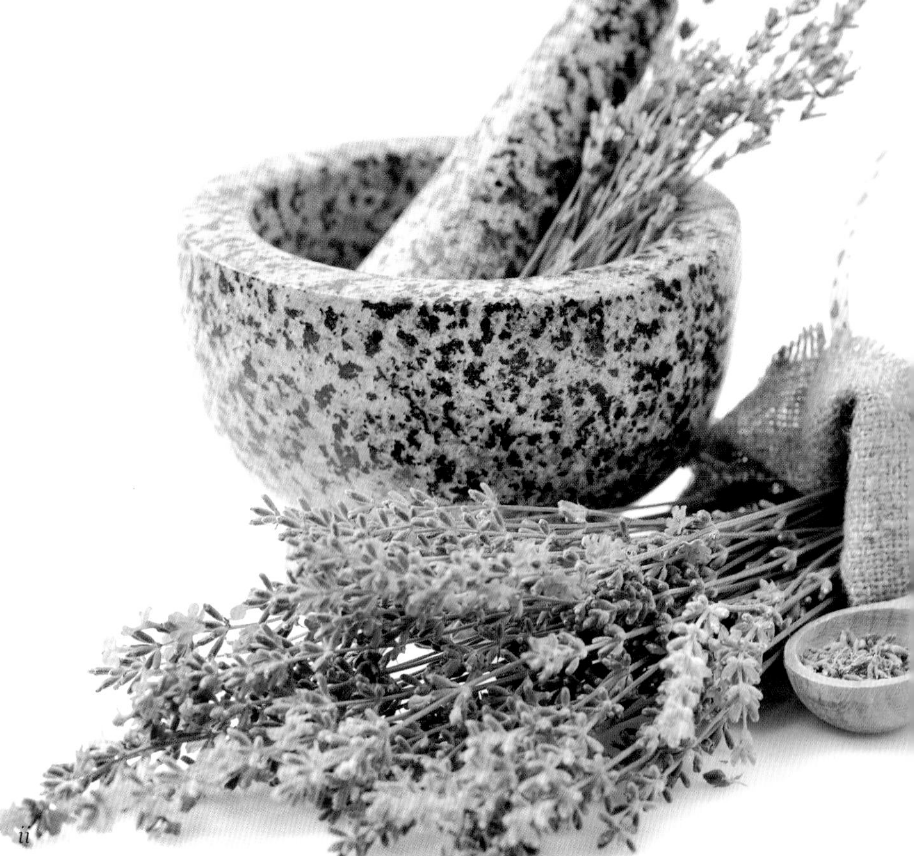

SEED TO SEAL™

Oils are as unique as the plants, ground, water, and air from which they come—even more so. How you cultivate, distill, test, and seal can make all the difference in the effectiveness of your oil. Young Living Essential Oils (YLEO) is the only company that truly provides a certified Seed to Seal™ guarantee. This means you can use them without fear.

Seed

Young Living selects the proper genus, species, and type for maximum potential. It's superior seeds that make superior plants.

Cultivate

This is about perfect growing and harvesting. Young Living uses the most organic, uncontaminated earth and water for pristine growing conditions. Timing is everything in ripening the most beneficial organic compounds in the plants. Even harvesting at specific times of the day can have a profound effect on the finished product. That's why YLEO takes everything into consideration to produce the most potent life-giving results. Young Living experts travel the world— exploring viability and inspecting all operations to ensure standards, quality and sustainability.

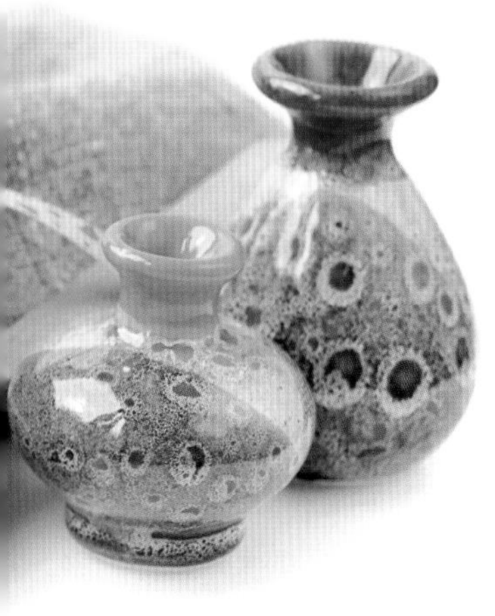

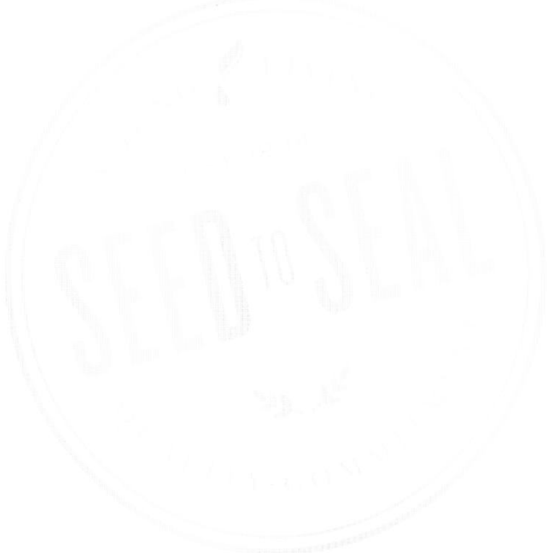

Distill

This is both an art and a science, and our personally controlled distilleries combine the best of modern and ancient techniques—steam, cold press, and resin-tapping—to produce the most compound-rich essential oils. These processes are proprietary, diverse, and innovative.

Test

Only the purest oils make the grade. Young Living personally tests for composition using FT-R spectroscopy, refractive index, specific gravity, optical rotation, gas chromatography, purity through ICP-MS, microbiological presence, peroxide value, flash point, and combustibility. These ensure not only that each bottle complies with any and all international standards, but also preserves the most organic bioactive compounds. But they don't stop there. Young Living guarantees consistent, verifiable quality by testing in third-party facilities as well.

Seal

Using state-of-the-art equipment, Young Living carefully seals each UV-protected bottle of essential oil in a clean-room facility for shipping to their members worldwide. It's single-source shipping at its best.

Seeing is Believing!

Young Living has eyes on every step of the process to ensure the purity of the finished products. Young Living is the only company in the world to have this kind of quality control. When you explore each essential oil, you are opening yourself up to a safe, organic, and vital addition to a healthy lifestyle.

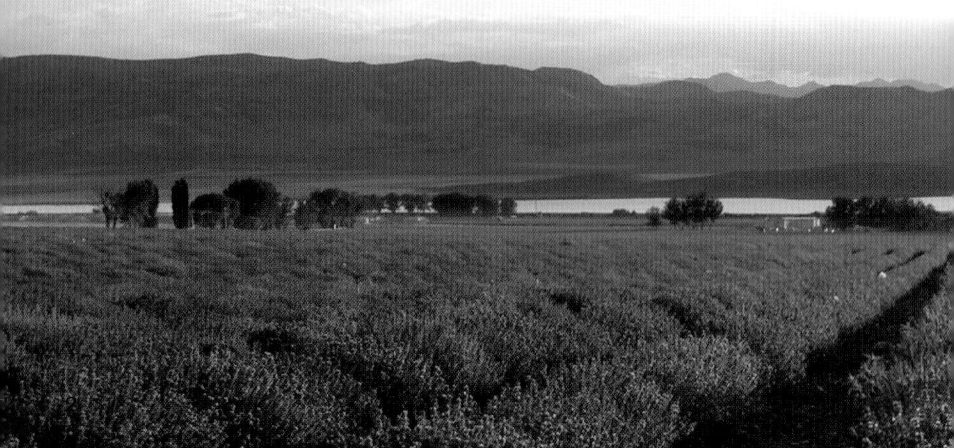

BASIC GUIDELINES

(Adapted from the Essential Oil Desk Reference, 6th Edition)

Because essential oils are so concentrated, they are powerful. That means you have to manage this power and use it with care. Here are some great guidelines to keep you and your family in the know. Remember, nothing can ever replace common sense. Always start gradually and patiently find what works best for you and your family members.

Storage

1. Always keep a bottle of a pure vegetable oil (e.g., V-6 Vegetable Oil Complex, olive oil, almond oil, coconut oil, or more fragrant massage oils such as Sensation, Relaxation, Ortho Ease, or Ortho Sport) handy when using essential oils. Vegetable oils will dilute essential oils if the essential oils cause discomfort or skin irritation.

2. Keep bottles of essential oils tightly closed and store them in a cool location away from light. If stored properly, essential oils will maintain their potency for many years.

3. Keep essential oils out of reach of children. Treat the oils as you would any product for therapeutic use. Children love the oils and will often go through an entire bottle in a very short time. They want to give massages and do the same things they see you do.

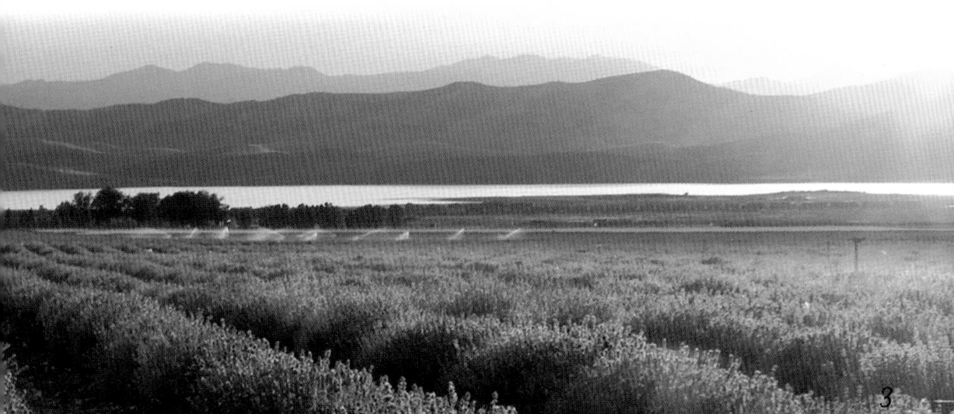

Usage

4. Essential oils rich in menthol (such as Peppermint) should not be used on the throat or neck area of children under 18 months of age.

5. Angelica, Bergamot, Grapefruit, Lemon, Orange, Tangerine, and other citrus oils are photosensitive and may cause a rash or dark pigmentation on skin exposed to direct sunlight or UV rays within 1–2 days after application.

6. Keep essential oils away from the eye area and never put them directly into ears. Do not handle contact lenses or rub eyes with essential oils on your fingers. Even in minute amounts, many essential oils may damage contacts and will irritate eyes.

7. Pregnant women should consult a health-care professional when starting any type of health program. Oils are safe to use, but one needs to use common sense. Follow the directions and dilute with V-6 Vegetable Oil Complex until you become familiar with the oils you are using. Many pregnant women have said that they feel a very positive response from the unborn child when the oils are applied on the skin, but that is each woman's individual experience.

8. Epileptics and those with high blood pressure should consult their health-care professional before using essential oils. Use extra caution with high ketone oils such as Basil, Rosemary, Sage, and Tansy oils.

9. People with allergies should test a small amount of oil on an area of sensitive skin, such as the inside of the upper arm, for 30 minutes before applying the oil on other areas of the body.

10. The bottoms of feet are safe locations to apply essential oils topically.

11. Direct inhalation of essential oils can be a deep and intensive application method, particularly for respiratory congestion and illness. However, this method should not be used more than 10–15 times throughout the day without consulting a health professional. Also, inhalation of essential oils is NOT recommended for those with asthmatic conditions.

12. Before taking GRAS (Generally Regarded As Safe) essential oils internally, test your reactions by diluting 1 drop of essential oil in 1 teaspoon of an oil-soluble liquid like Blue Agave, Yacon Syrup, olive oil, coconut oil, or rice milk. If you intend to consume more than a few drops of diluted essential oil per day, we recommend first consulting a health professional.

13. Be aware that reactions to essential oils, both topically and orally, can be delayed as long as 2–3 days.

14. Add 1–3 drops of undiluted essential oils directly to bath water. If more essential oil is desired, mix the oil first into bath salts or a bath gel base before adding to the bath water. Generally, never use more than 10 drops of essential oils in one bath. When essential oils are put directly into bath water without a dispersing agent, they can cause serious discomfort on sensitive skin because the essential oils tend to float, undiluted, on top of the water.

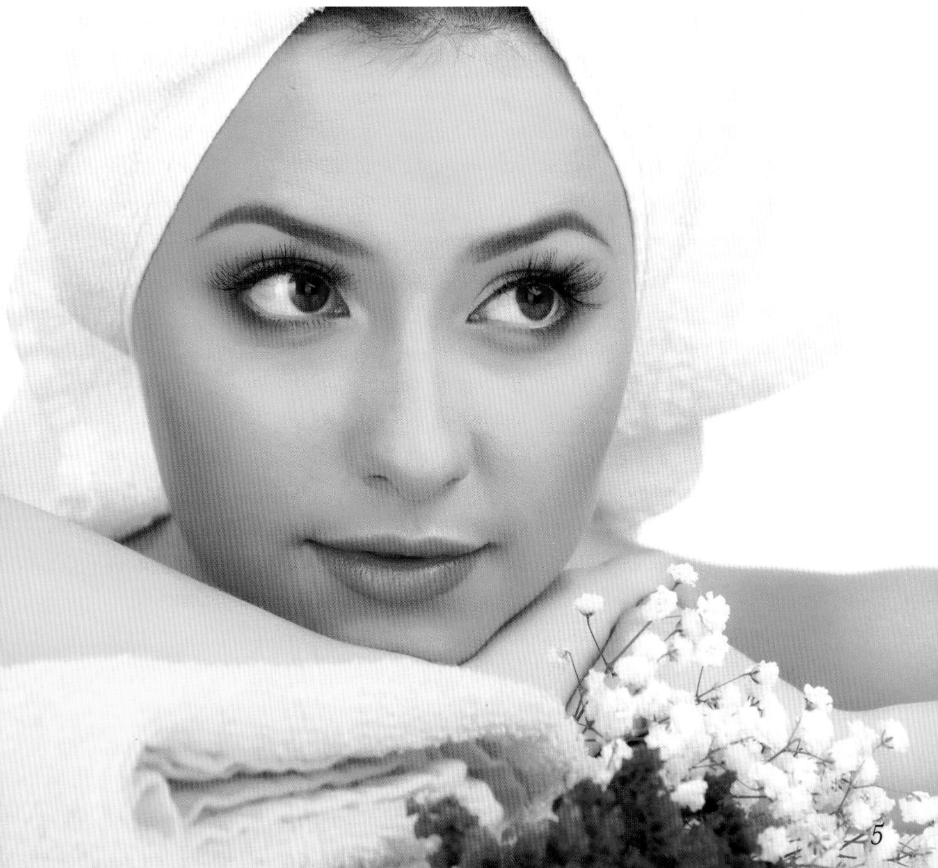

Chemical Sensitivities and Allergies

Occasionally, people with high skin sensitivity, who begin using ultra-pure essential oils, will experience rashes or reactions. This might happen when using an undiluted spice, conifer, or citrus oil. Or, the oil may interact with residues of synthetic, petroleum-based, personal-care products that have leached into the skin.

When using essential oils on a daily basis, you'll want to avoid personal-care products containing ammonium or hydrocarbon-based chemicals. This is a must. Be on the watch for quaternary compounds such as quaternariums and polyquaternariums. These chemicals can be fatal if ingested, especially benzalkonium chloride, which, unfortunately, is used in many personal-care products on the market.

Other chemicals such as aluminum compounds, FD&C colors, formaldehyde, parabens, talc, thimerosal, mercury, and titanium dioxide, just to name a few, can all be toxic to your body. You'll want to avoid those! These compounds are fairly common in hand creams, mouthwashes, shampoos, antiperspirants, after-shave lotions, and hair-care products.

The other ones you'll want to watch out for are sodium lauryl sulfate, propylene glycol (found in almost everything from toothpaste to shampoo), and aluminum salts (found in most deodorants).

Above all, avoid the synthetic fragrances that are everywhere, including methylene chloride, methyl isobutyl ketone, and methyl ethyl ketone. These are not only toxic, but they can also react with some compounds in natural essential oils. The result can be a severe case of dermatitis or even septicemia (blood poisoning).

After they are absorbed, these chemicals can become trapped in the fatty subdermal layers of skin, where they can leach into the bloodstream. They can remain trapped for several months or years until a topical substance, like an essential oil, starts to move them from their resting place and cause them to come out of the skin in an uncomfortable way. Besides skin irritation, you could experience nausea, headaches, and other slight temporary effects during this detoxifying process. Even in small concentrations, these chemicals and synthetic compounds are toxic and are a threat to your health.

If you have a sensitive reaction, you can always reduce the amount

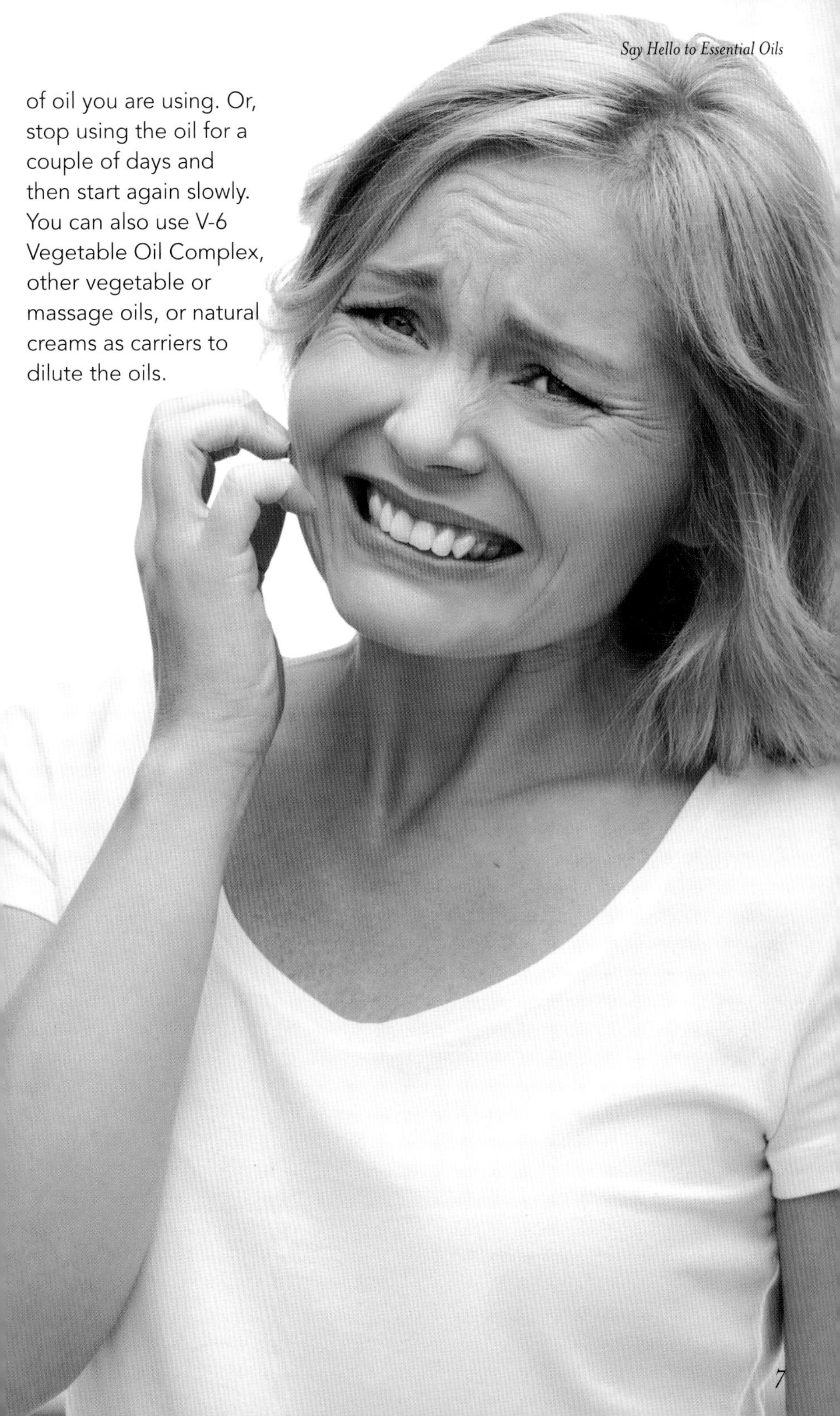

of oil you are using. Or, stop using the oil for a couple of days and then start again slowly. You can also use V-6 Vegetable Oil Complex, other vegetable or massage oils, or natural creams as carriers to dilute the oils.

BEFORE YOU START

(Adapted from the Essential Oil Desk Reference, 6th Edition)

Always skin test an essential oil before using it. Everyone is different. Your body is unique, so apply oils to a small area first. Apply one oil or blend at a time. When layering oils that are new to you, allow enough time (3-5 minutes) for the body to respond before applying a second oil.

Use a small amount when you apply essential oils to your skin—especially in areas that may carry residue from cosmetics, personal-care products, soaps, and cleansers containing synthetic chemicals. Some of them—especially petroleum-based chemicals—can penetrate and remain in the skin and fatty tissues for days or even weeks after use.

Essential oils may work against such chemicals and toxins built up in the body and bring them to the surface. If you have this kind of an experience using essential oils, reduce or stop using them for a few days and start an internal cleansing program before you start again. It's a great idea to double your water intake and keep flushing those toxins out of your body.

You may also want to try the following alternatives to a detoxification program to determine the cause of the problem:

- Dilute 1–3 drops of essential oil in 1/2 teaspoon of V-6 Vegetable Oil Complex, massage oil, or any pure vegetable oil such as almond, coconut, or olive. More dilution may be needed.
- Reduce the number of oils used at any time.
- Use single oils or oil blends one at a time.
- Reduce the amount of oil used.
- Reduce the frequency of application.
- Drink more purified or distilled water.
- Ask your health-care professional to monitor detoxification.
- Test the diluted essential oil on a small patch of skin for 30 minutes. If any redness or irritation results, dilute the area immediately with a pure vegetable or massage oil and then cleanse with soap and water.
- If skin irritation or other uncomfortable side effects persist, discontinue using the oil on that location and apply the oils on the bottoms of the feet.

You may also want to avoid using products that contain the following ingredients to eliminate potential problems:

- Cosmetics, deodorants, and skin-care products containing aluminum, petrochemicals, or other synthetic ingredients.
- Perms, hair colors or dyes, hair sprays, or gels containing synthetic chemicals; shampoos, toothpastes, mouthwashes, and soaps containing synthetic chemicals such as sodium laurel sulfate, propylene glycol, or lead acetate.
- Garden sprays, paints, detergents, and cleansers containing toxic chemicals and solvents.

You can use many essential oils anywhere on the body except on the eyes and in the ears. Other oils may irritate certain sensitive tissues. See recommended dilution on the bottles to be sure.

Keep "hot" oils such as Oregano, Cinnamon, Thyme, Eucalyptus, Mountain Savory, Lemon, and Orange essential oils or blends such as Thieves, PanAway, Relieve It, and Exodus II out of children's reach. These types of oils should always be diluted for both children and adults.

Children need to be taught how to use the oils so that they understand the safety issue. If a child or infant swallows an essential oil, do the following:

- Seek immediate emergency medical attention, if necessary.
- Give the child milk, cream, yogurt, or another safe, oil-soluble liquid to drink.

NOTE: If your body pH is low, your body will be acidic; therefore, you could also have less of a response or perhaps a minimal negative reaction to the oils.

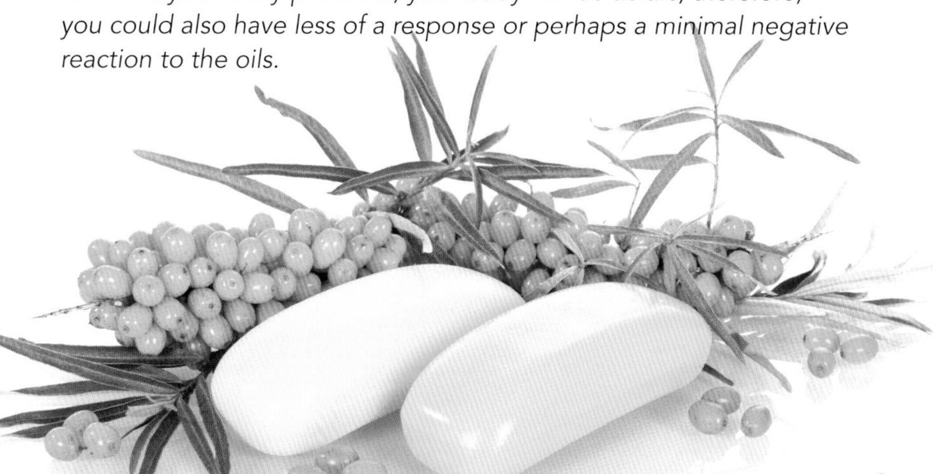

TOPICAL APPLICATION

(Adapted from the Essential Oil Desk Reference, 6th Edition)

Many oils are safe to apply directly to the skin. Lavender is safe to use on children without dilution. But you have to be sure the essential oil you are using is not lavandin, commercially labeled as lavender or genetically altered lavender. When applying most other essential oils on children, dilute the oils with carrier oil. For dilution, add 15–30 drops of essential oil to 1 oz. of quality carrier oil.

Carrier oils such as V-6 Vegetable Oil Complex extend essential oils and provide more efficient use. When massaging, the vegetable oil helps lubricate the skin.

When you start applying, depending on which oil you use, you may want to test for skin sensitivity by dabbing the oil first on the bottoms of the feet. See the Vita Flex foot charts to identify areas of best application. Start by applying 3–6 drops of a single oil or blend, spreading it over the bottom of each foot, focusing on the area of the foot that corresponds to the rest of the body.

When applying essential oils to yourself, use 1–2 drops of oil on 2–3 locations 2 times a day. Gradually increase to 4 times a day, if needed. Apply the oil and allow it to absorb for 2–3 minutes before applying another oil or before getting dressed to avoid staining your clothes.

As a general rule, when applying oils to yourself or another person for the first time, do not apply more than two single oils or blends at one time.

When mixing essential oil blends or diluting essential oils in a carrier oil, it is best to use glass or earthenware containers, rather than plastic. Many plastics will react—even dissolve—when put in contact with essential oils. Plastic particles can leach into the oil and then into the skin once it is applied. If you must use a plastic container, look for HDPE or PETE (recycling symbols 1 or 2), because these are less likely to react.

Before applying oils, wash hands thoroughly with soap and water.

Massage

Start by applying 2 drops of a single oil or blend on the skin and massaging it in. If you are working on a large area, such as the back, mix 1–3 drops of the selected essential oil into 1 teaspoon of pure carrier oil such as V-6 Vegetable Oil Complex, a massage oil, or any other oil of your choice such as jojoba, almond, coconut, olive, and/or grape seed.

Keep in mind that many massage oils such as olive, almond, jojoba, or wheat germ oil may stain some fabrics.

Acupuncture

Licensed acupuncturists can dramatically increase the effectiveness of acupuncture by using essential oils.

To start, place several drops of essential oil into the palm of your hand and dip the acupuncture needle tip into the oil before inserting it into the person. You can premix several oils in your hand if you wish to use more than one oil.

Acupressure

When performing an acupressure treatment, apply 1–3 drops of essential oil to the acupressure point with your finger. Using an auricular probe with a slender point to dispense oil, may enhance the application.

Start by pressing firmly and then releasing. Avoid applying pressure to any particular pressure point too long. You may continue along the acupressure points and meridians or use the reflexology or Vita Flex points as well. Once you have completed small point stimulations, massage the general area with the essential oil.

Warm Compress

For deeper penetration, use a warm compress after applying essential oils. Completely soak the cloth or towel by placing it in comfortably hot water. By the time you wring out the cloth and shake it, it will be a nice, warm temperature to be placed on the location. Then cover the cloth loosely with a dry towel or blanket to seal in the heat. Leave the cloth on for 15-30 minutes. Remove the cloth immediately if there is any discomfort.

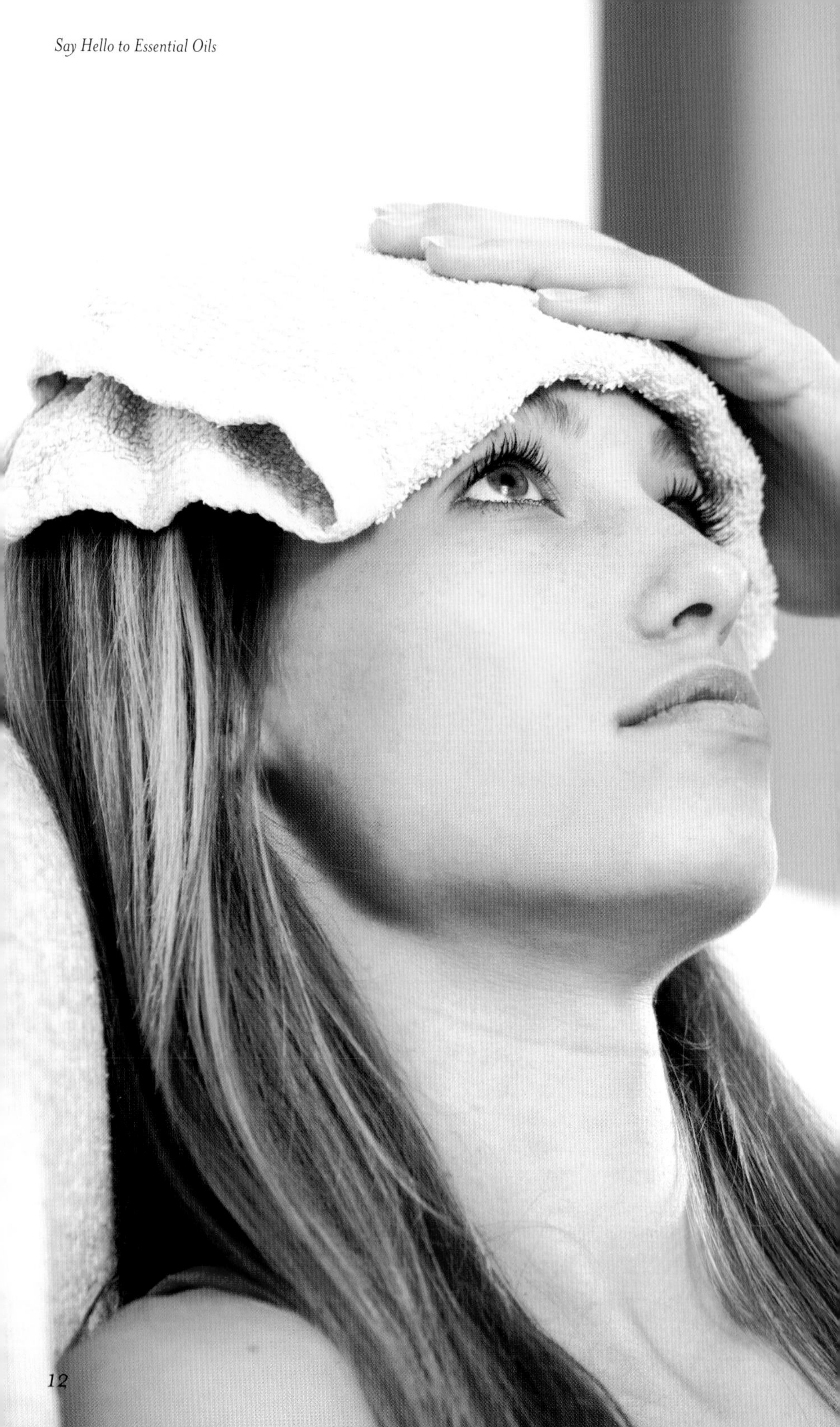

Cold Packs

Apply essential oils on the location, followed by cold water or ice packs when treating inflamed or swollen tissues. Frozen packages of peas or corn make excellent ice packs that will mold to the contours of the body part and will not leak. Keep the cold pack on until the swelling diminishes. For neurological problems, always use cold packs, never hot packs.

Layering

This technique consists of applying multiple oils one at a time. For example, rub Marjoram over a sore muscle, massage it into the tissue gently until the area is dry, and then apply a second oil such as Peppermint until the oil is absorbed and the skin is dry. Then layer on the third oil, such as Basil, and continue massaging.

Making a Compress

- Rub 1–3 drops on the location, diluted or neat, depending on the oil used and the skin sensitivity at that location.
- Cover the location with a hot, damp towel.
- Cover the moist towel with a dry towel for 10–30 minutes, depending on individual need.

As the oil penetrates the skin, you may experience a warming or even a burning sensation, especially in areas where the greatest benefits occur. If burning becomes uncomfortable, apply V-6 Vegetable Oil Complex, a massage oil, or any pure vegetable oil such as olive, coconut, or almond to the location.

A second type of application is very mild and is great for children or those with sensitive skin:

- Place 5-15 drops of essential oil into a basin filled with warm water.
- Water temperature should be approximately 100° F (38° C), unless the patient suffers neurological conditions; in that case, use cool water.
- Vigorously agitate the water and let it stand for 1 minute.
- Place a dry face cloth on top of the water to soak up oils that have floated to the surface.
- Wring out the water and apply the cloth on the location. To seal in the warmth, cover the location with a thick towel for 15–30 minutes.

Bath

Adding essential oils to bath water is challenging because oil does not mix with water. For even dispersion, mix 5–10 drops of essential oil in 1/4 cup of Epsom salts or bath gel base and then put the cup under a running faucet and gradually add water. This method will help the oils disperse in the bath evenly and prevent stronger oils from stinging sensitive areas.

You can also use premixed bath gels and shampoos containing essential oils as a liquid soap in the shower or bath. Lather down with the bath gel, let it soak in, and then rinse. To maximize benefits, leave the soap or shampoo on the skin or scalp for several minutes to allow the essential oils to penetrate.

You can create your own aromatic bath gels by placing 5–15 drops of essential oil in 1/2 oz. of an unscented bath gel base and then add to the bath water as described above.

Shower

Essential oils can be added to Epsom salts and used in the shower. Some shower heads or sprayers can work with your natural shower to distribute the oils in "softer" water. This allows essential oils to not only make contact with the skin but also diffuses the fragrance of the oils into the air. These kinds of fixtures can hold approximately 1/4 to 1/2 cup of bath salts.
Or, you can always place a few drops of oil on the edge of your shower floor. As you shower under the hot water, the natural steam will carry the aroma all around your bathroom. It's a wonderful way to start the day.

How to Enhance the Benefits of Topical Application

The longer essential oils stay in contact with the skin, the more likely they are to be absorbed. The A•R•T Night Reconstructor or A•R•T Day Activator lotions, Sandalwood Moisture Cream, or Boswellia Wrinkle Cream may be layered on top of the essential oils to reduce evaporation of the oils and enhance penetration. This may also help seal and protect cuts and wounds. Do not use ointments on burns until they are at least three days old; however, LavaDerm Cooling Mist spray may be used immediately to provide comforting relief for minor burns, abrasions, dryness, and other skin irritations.

DIFFUSING

Diffused oils alter the structure of molecules that create odors, rather than just masking them. They also increase oxygen availability, produce negative ions, and release natural ozone. Many essential oils such as Lemongrass, Orange, Grapefruit, Melaleuca Alternifolia—Tea Tree, Eucalyptus Globulus, Lavender, Frankincense, and Lemon, along with essential oil blends (Purification, Melrose, and Thieves), are extremely effective for eliminating and destroying airborne germs and bacteria.

A cold-air diffuser is designed to atomize a microfine mist of essential oils, lifting them gently into the air, where they can remain suspended for several hours. Unlike aroma lamps or candles, a diffuser disperses essential oils without heating or burning, which can render the oil therapeutically less beneficial and even create toxic compounds.

Research shows that cold-air diffusing certain oils may:

- Reduce unpleasant odors.
- May help provide uplifting, fresh, clear, and relaxing environment.
- Help support healthy weight management*.
- Help support concentration, alertness, and mental clarity*.
- Help support healthy systems of the body*.
- Help support healthy balance*.
- Help support a positive emotional environment.

Guidelines for Diffusing

- Check the viscosity or thickness of the oil you want to diffuse. If the oil has too much natural wax and is too thick, it could plug the diffuser and make cleaning difficult.
- Start by diffusing oils for 15–30 minutes a day. As you become accustomed to the oils and recognize their effects, you may increase the diffusing time to 1–2 hours per day.
- By connecting your diffuser to a timer, you can gain better control over the length and duration of diffusing. For some respiratory conditions, you may diffuse the oils the entire night.

** These statements have not been evaluated by the Food and Drug Administration. Young Living products are not intended to diagnose, cure, treat, or prevent any disease.*

- Do not use more than one blend at a time in a diffuser, as this may alter the smell and the therapeutic benefit. However, a single oil may be added to a blend when diffusing.
- Place the diffuser high in the room so that the oil mist falls through the air and removes the odor-causing substances.
- If you want to wash the diffuser before using a different oil blend, use Thieves Household Cleaner with warm water or any natural soap and warm water.
- If you do not have a diffuser, you can add several drops of essential oil to a spray bottle with 1 cup purified water and shake. You can use this to mist your entire house, workplace, or car.

Air Freshener Oil Recipe:

- 20 drops Lavender
- 10 drops Lemon
- 6 drops Bergamot
- 5 drops Lime
- 5 drops Grapefruit

Diffuse neat or mix with 1 cup of distilled water in a spray bottle; shake well before spraying.

Other Ways to Diffuse Oils

- Add your favorite essential oils to cedar chips to make your own potpourri.
- Put scented cedar chips in your closets or drawers to deodorize them.
- Sprinkle a few drops of conifer essential oils such as Spruce, Fir (all varieties), Cedar, or Pine onto logs in the fireplace. As the logs burn, they will disperse an evergreen smell. This method has no therapeutic benefit, however.
- Put essential oils on cotton balls or tissues and place them in your car, home, work, or hotel heating or air conditioning vents.
- Put a few drops of oil in a bowl or pan of water and set it on a warm stove.
- On a damp cloth, sprinkle a few drops of one of your purifying essential oils and place the cloth near an intake duct of your heating and cooling system so that the air can carry the aroma throughout your home.

Humidifier and Vaporizer

Essential oils make ideal additions to humidifiers or vaporizers. Always check the viscosity of the oil, because if it is too thick, it could plug the humidifier or make it difficult to clean. The following singles and blends are great to diffuse.

Singles: Idaho Balsam Fir, Frankincense, Sacred Frankincense, Peppermint, Lemon, Eucalyptus Radiata, Melaleuca Alternifolia, Lavender, Ylang Ylang, and many others of your choice
Blends: Purification, Thieves, Raven, Melrose, Joy, RutaVaLa, The Gift, White Angelica, Sacred Mountain, and many others of your choice

NOTE: Test the oil before diffusing it in the vaporizer or humidifier; some essential oils may damage the plastic parts of vaporizers.

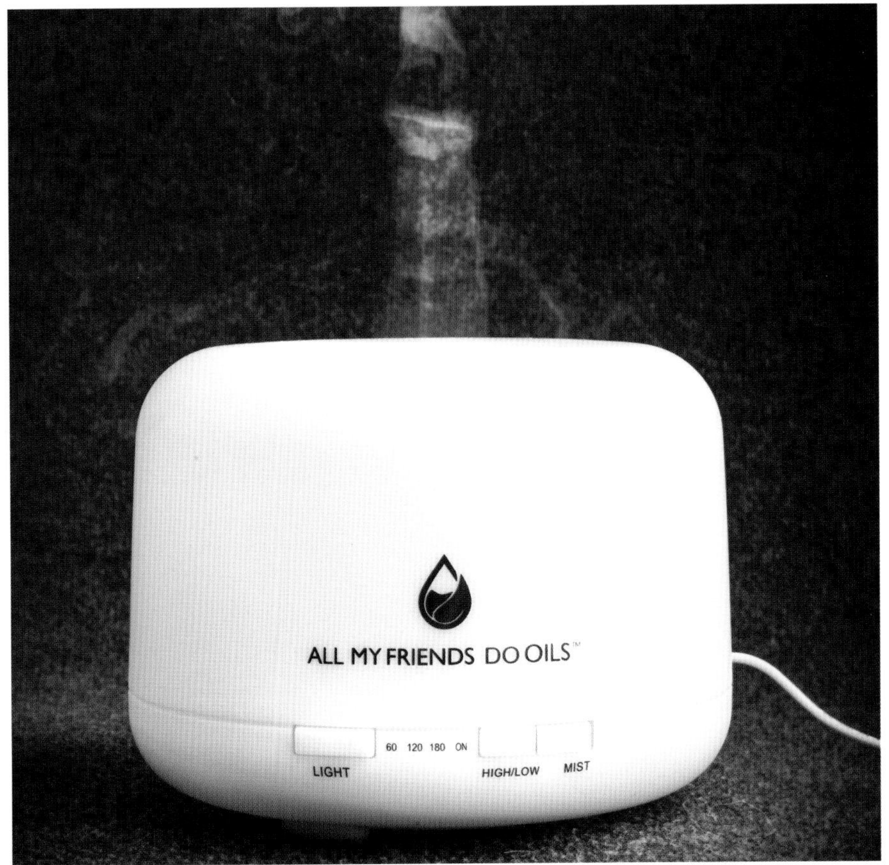

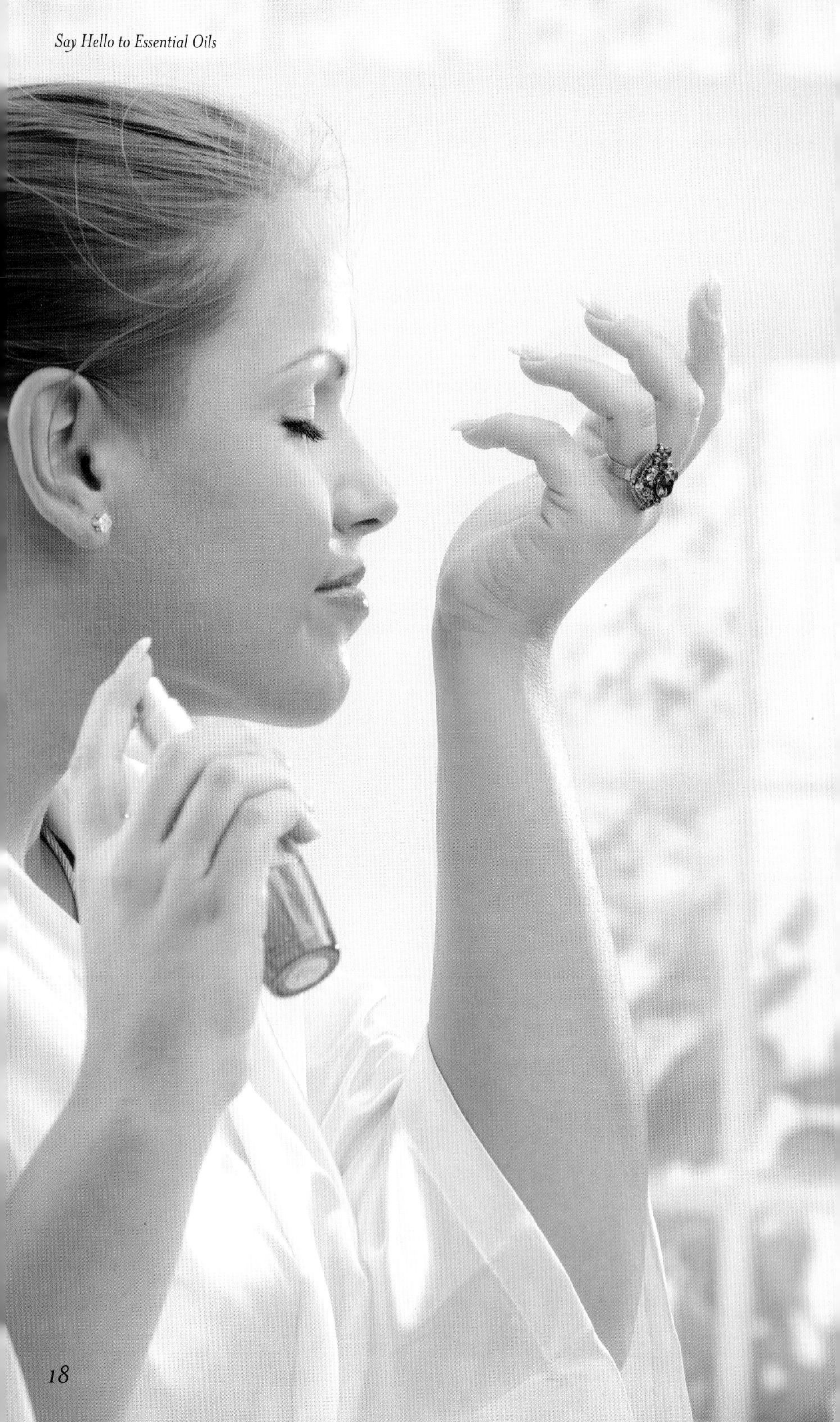

OTHER USES

Direct Inhalation

- Place 2 or more drops into the palm of your left hand and rub clockwise with the flat palm of your right hand. Cup your hands together over your nose and mouth and inhale deeply. (Do not touch your eyes!)
- Add several drops of an essential oil to a bowl of hot (not boiling) water. Inhale the steaming vapors that rise from the bowl. To increase the intensity of the oil vapors inhaled, drape a towel over your head and the bowl before inhaling.
- Apply oils to a cotton ball or tissue (do not use synthetic fibers or fabric) and place it in the air vent of your car.
- Inhale directly.

Indirect or Subtle Inhalation

(Wearing as a perfume or cologne)

- Rub 2 or more drops of oil on your chest, neck, upper sternum, wrists, or under your nose and ears, and enjoy the fragrance throughout the day.
- There are many necklaces with different types of vessels hanging on them into which you can pour a particular oil to use throughout the day.
- There are clay-type medallions to hang around your neck or fasten with a clip on your clothing onto which you can put a few oil drops to give off a gentle fragrance the entire day.

COPAIBA VITALITY™

Aromatic · Topical

NATURAL CONSTITUENTS

Alpha-copaene, Alpha-Humulene, Beta-Caryophyllene, Delta-Cadinene, Elta-Elemene, Gamma-Elemene, Germacrene D, Trans-Alpha-Bergamotene

This unique oil comes from the Brazilian copaiba tree resin. Its sweet, rich aroma imparts an positive grounding emotional effect. The high levels of beta-caryophyllene may account for its potentially calming effects. Use it before, during, and after workouts to support general wellness.

BEST RESULTS

- Add to a clear vegetable capsule to take daily as part of your health regimen.
- Add 1-2 drops to herbal tea for a "balsamic" flavor.
- Add 1-2 drops to white vinegar to create a more complex "woodsy" flavor.
- Add 1-2 drops to butter and whip together to create a tasty herbal topping.

BEST USES

- Apply to chest and neck.
- Fresh, comforting aroma promotes a calming effect.
- Diffuse to create a tranquil and serene aromatic environment.

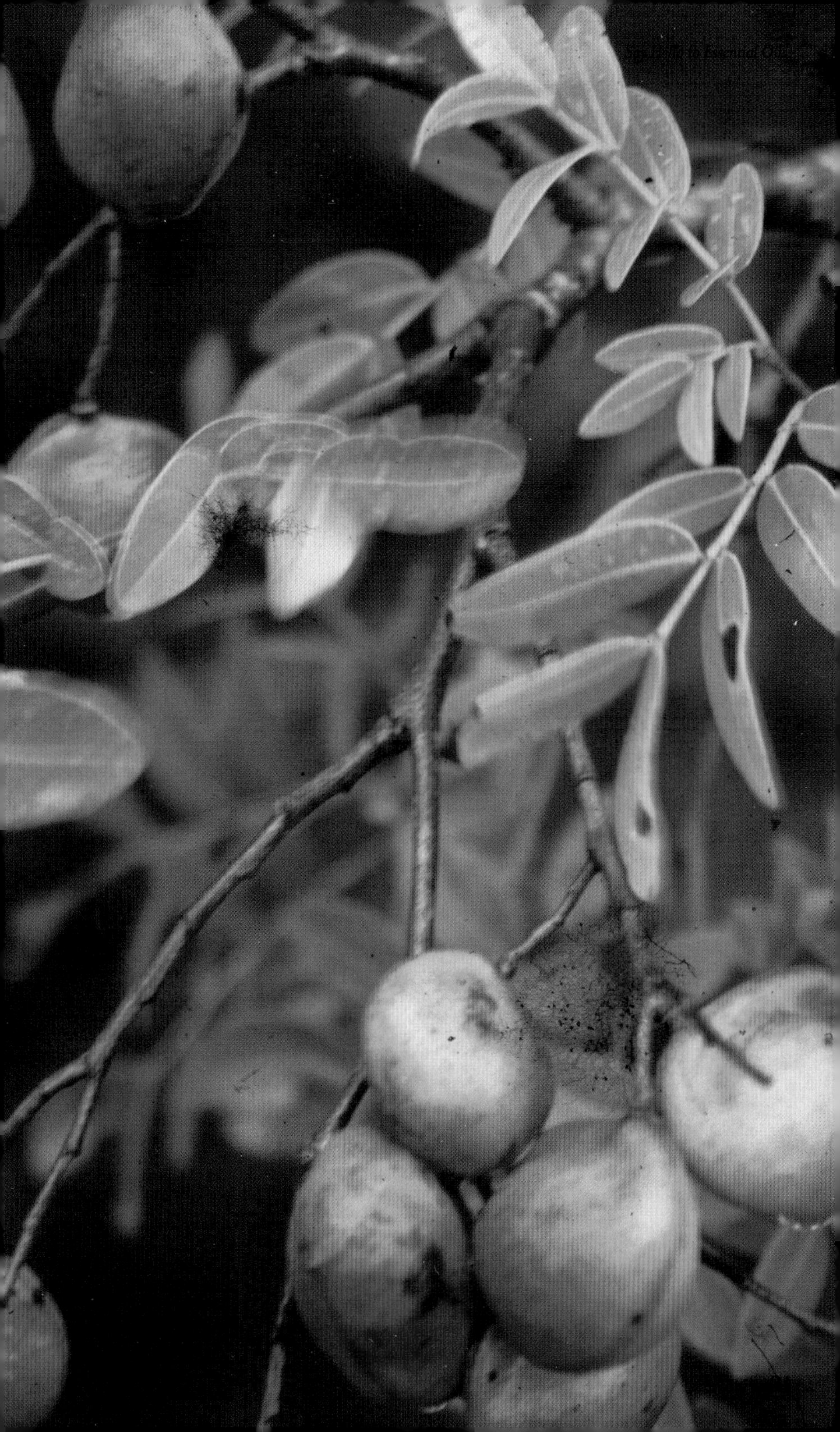

DIGIZE VITALITY™

Aromatic · Topical

Contains:
Tarragon · Ginger
Peppermint
Juniper · Fennel
Lemongrass
Anise · Patchouli

NATURAL CONSTITUENTS

Limonene, Menthol, Menthone

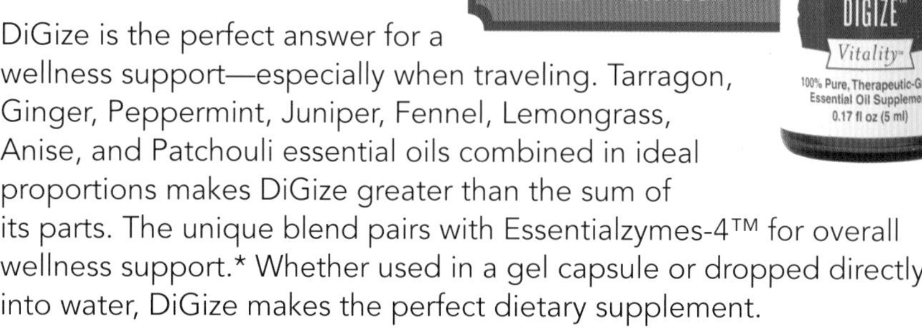

DiGize is the perfect answer for a wellness support—especially when traveling. Tarragon, Ginger, Peppermint, Juniper, Fennel, Lemongrass, Anise, and Patchouli essential oils combined in ideal proportions makes DiGize greater than the sum of its parts. The unique blend pairs with Essentialzymes-4™ for overall wellness support.* Whether used in a gel capsule or dropped directly into water, DiGize makes the perfect dietary supplement.

BEST RESULTS

- Add 1-2 drops to your favorite organic almond, soy, or cow's milk.
- Add 1-2 drops to your favorite organic smoothie.
- Add 1-2 drops to a vegetable gelatin capsule.
- Add 1-2 drops to your favorite salad dressing.

BEST USES

- Support healthy digestion by taking as a dietary supplement in a capsule.
- Combine with Essentialzymes-4™ and use after meals to support your healthy regimen.*
- Add 2 drops DiGize and 1 drop Peppermint to purified water for a great infusion.
- Ancient Egyptians revered the properties of Fennel, one of the constituent oils in DiGize.
- Help support your health during international travel by adding 1-2 drops to foods and beverages or a capsule.
- Add 2-3 drops to hot water and honey for a great tasting beverage.

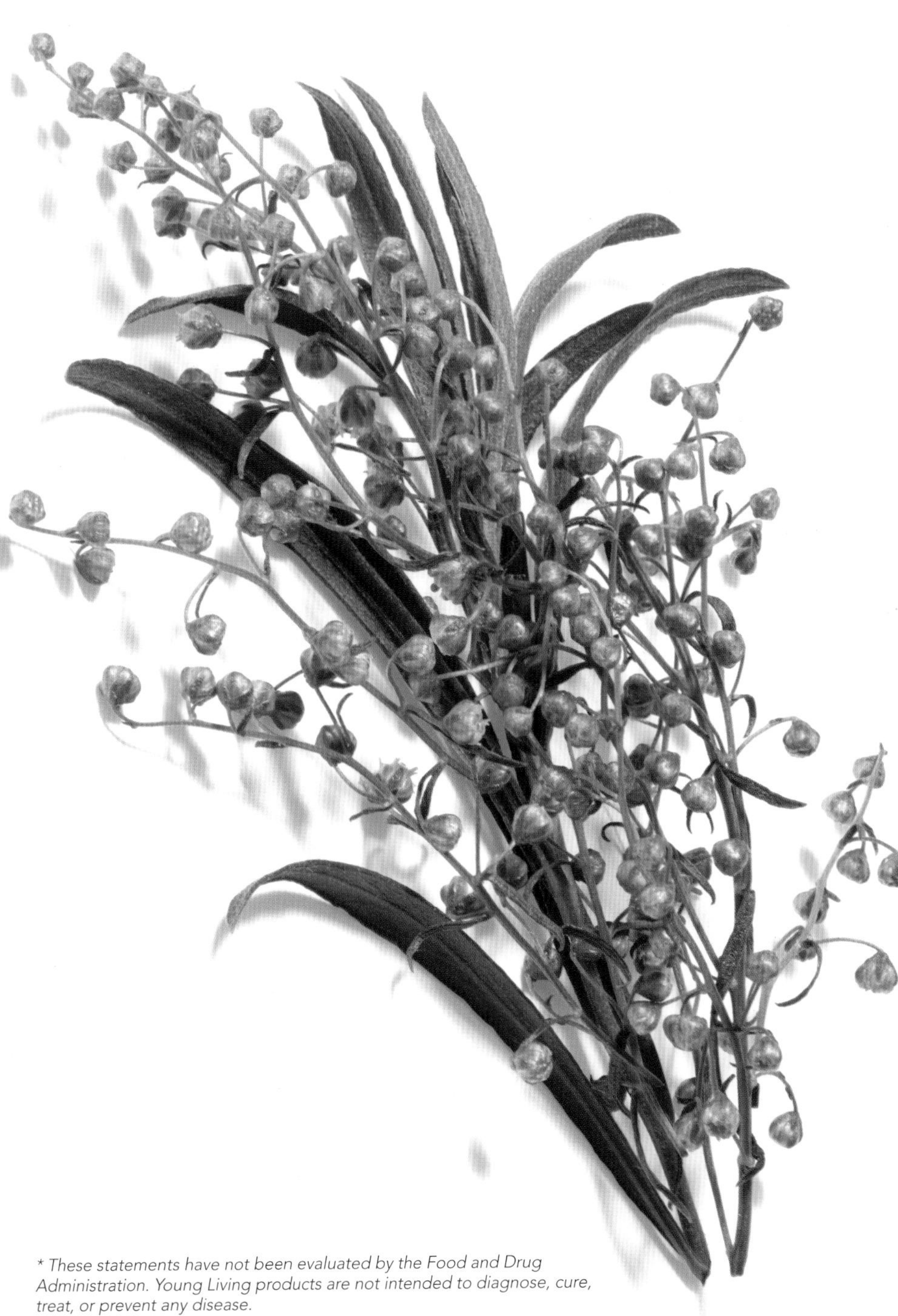

* These statements have not been evaluated by the Food and Drug Administration. Young Living products are not intended to diagnose, cure, treat, or prevent any disease.

FRANKINCENSE

Aromatic · Topical

NATURAL CONSTITUENTS

Alpha-Pinene, Limonene, Sabinene, Myrcene, Beta-Caryphyllene, Alpha-Thujene, Incensole

ORAC: 630 μTE/100g

Frankincense (boswellia carteri) was considered more valuable than gold in ancient times and used by ancient cultures to ease many conditions. Scientists have studied it to examine antitumoral, immunostimulant, antidepressant and muscle relaxing potential—as well as potential effects on the limbic system of the brain, the hypothalamus, pineal gland, and pituitary gland.

Frankincense is perfect for boosting spirituality. Its earthy, grounding fragrance draws focus and clarity. The natural constituent alpha-pinene makes Frankincense a key ingredient in many blends. It's also great for post-activity rejuvenation. Its unique properties make it a wonderful moisturizer and skin conditioner.

BEST USES

- Diffuse during meditation for resolve and intention.
- Combine 1-5 drops with V-6™. Vegetable Oil Complex and massage muscles after exercise.
- Combine 1-2 drops with your favorite moisturizer to complement healthy-looking skin.

** These statements have not been evaluated by the Food and Drug Administration. Young Living products are not intended to diagnose, cure, treat, or prevent any disease.*

BEST RESULTS

- Get your game on: use 1-2 drops on temples and back of neck to help maintain concentration.
- Elevate your spiritual experiences: diffuse in your home or office.
- Support your glowing skin: add 1-2 drops to your daily application of lotion.
- Highlight your radiant skin: add 1-2 drops to your night cream.
- Enhance yoga: diffuse during your yoga routine.
- Follow up your workout: enjoy a post-activity massage using 1-2 drops in 1 teaspoon of carrier oil.
- Uplift your spirits: inhale deeply, directly from the bottle.
- Help skin stay smooth: add 10 drops to 1 tablespoon of carrier oil. Use as a daily moisturizer.
- Enhance your bath: add 10 drops to 1 tablespoon of carrier oil. Combine with Epsom salts and enjoy.
- Sparkling nails: add 2 drops to 1 teaspoon of coconut oil and massage into nails and nail beds for dazzling effects.
- Work smarter: diffuse for 15 minutes while focusing on creating solutions to work challenges.
- Stay positive: give your brainstorming session that ultimate kick by diffusing for 15 minutes when you start capturing ideas.

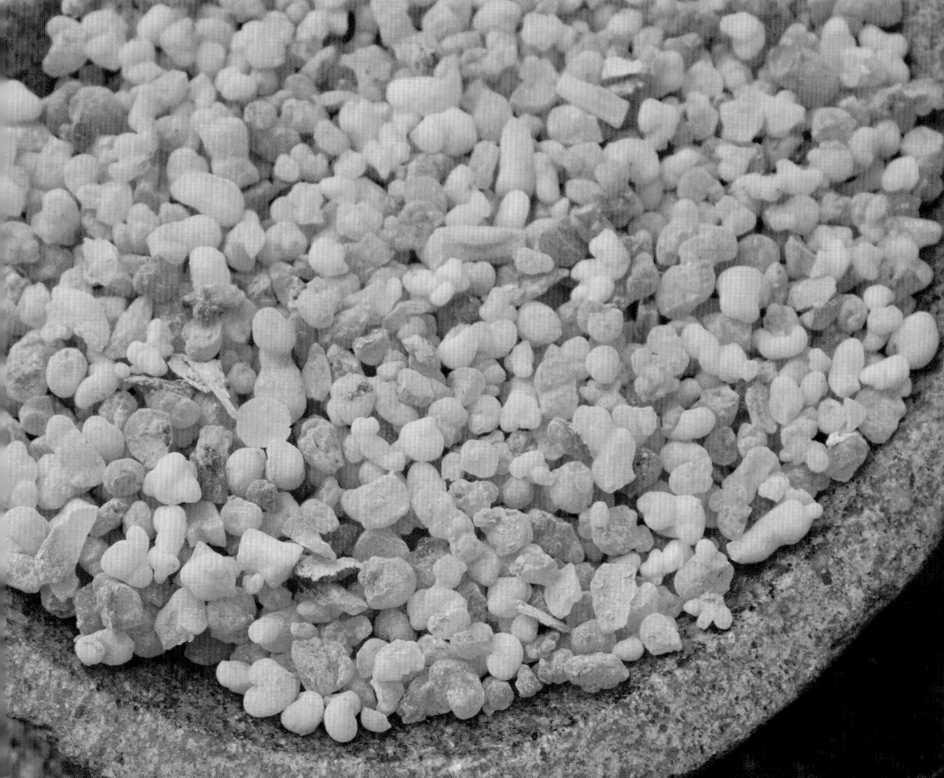

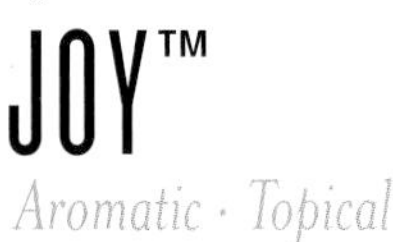

JOY™

Aromatic · Topical

NATURAL CONSTITUENTS

Citronellol, Geraniol, Citronellyl Formate, Linalool

Contains:
Bergamot · Ylang Ylang
Geranium · Lemon
Coriander
Tangerine · Jasmine
Roman Chamomile
Palmarosa · Rose

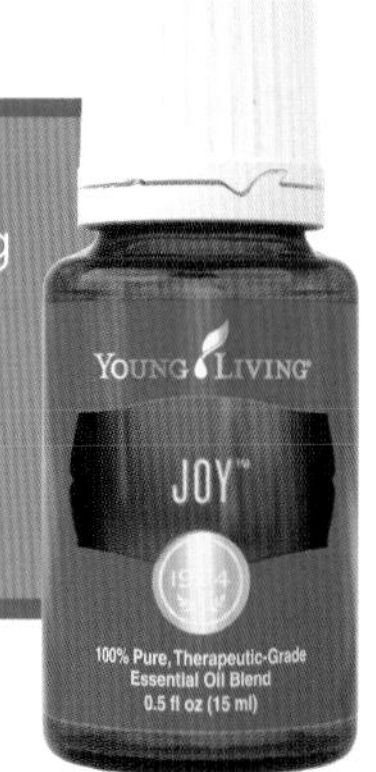

Joy™ is an emotionally balanced blend of Lemon, Mandarin, Bergamot, Ylang Ylang, Rose, Rosewood, Geranium, Palmarosa, Roman Chamomile, and Jasmine. Joy is a therapeutic-grade essential oil blend designed to uplift, help overcome frustration, and brighten your day.

Joy's sprightly, bold blend of jubilant essential oils, this euphoric blend of harmonizing essential oils inspires romance, bliss, and warmth when diffused. Add it to your favorite moisturizer or bath base for a vibrant, exhilarating experience.

BEST RESULTS

- Uplifting boost: rub a drop over the heart and on the bottom of each foot.
- Frustration: rub a drop over the heart and on the bottom of each foot.
- Inspiration: put a drop on the tip of the nose.
- Perfume: wear a drop behind each ear.
- Aftershave: rub a drop between your palms and then spread over the face and neck.
- Body/leg shaving: rub a drop between your palms and then spread over the shaved areas.
- Fragrance: sprinkle a few drops into potpourri.
- Poor circulation: rub 2 drops on areas of the body with poor circulation to improve blood flow.
- Deodorant: put 2 drops on the armpit area.
- Spark the romance: rub 2 drops on the heart and feet.
- Sweeten laundry: put 2 drops on a wet cloth and put in the dryer for great smelling clothes.
- Relaxing bath: mix 1-2 drops with YL Bath Gel Base in warm water for a relaxing bath.

BEST RESULTS

- The aroma encourages a romantic, aromatic environment.
- Diffuse for a warm, ebullient atmosphere.
- Add to your favorite lotion or moisturizer to support luminous skin.
- Add to a relaxing bath to help you unwind.
- Evokes romance and intimacy when worn as cologne or perfume.

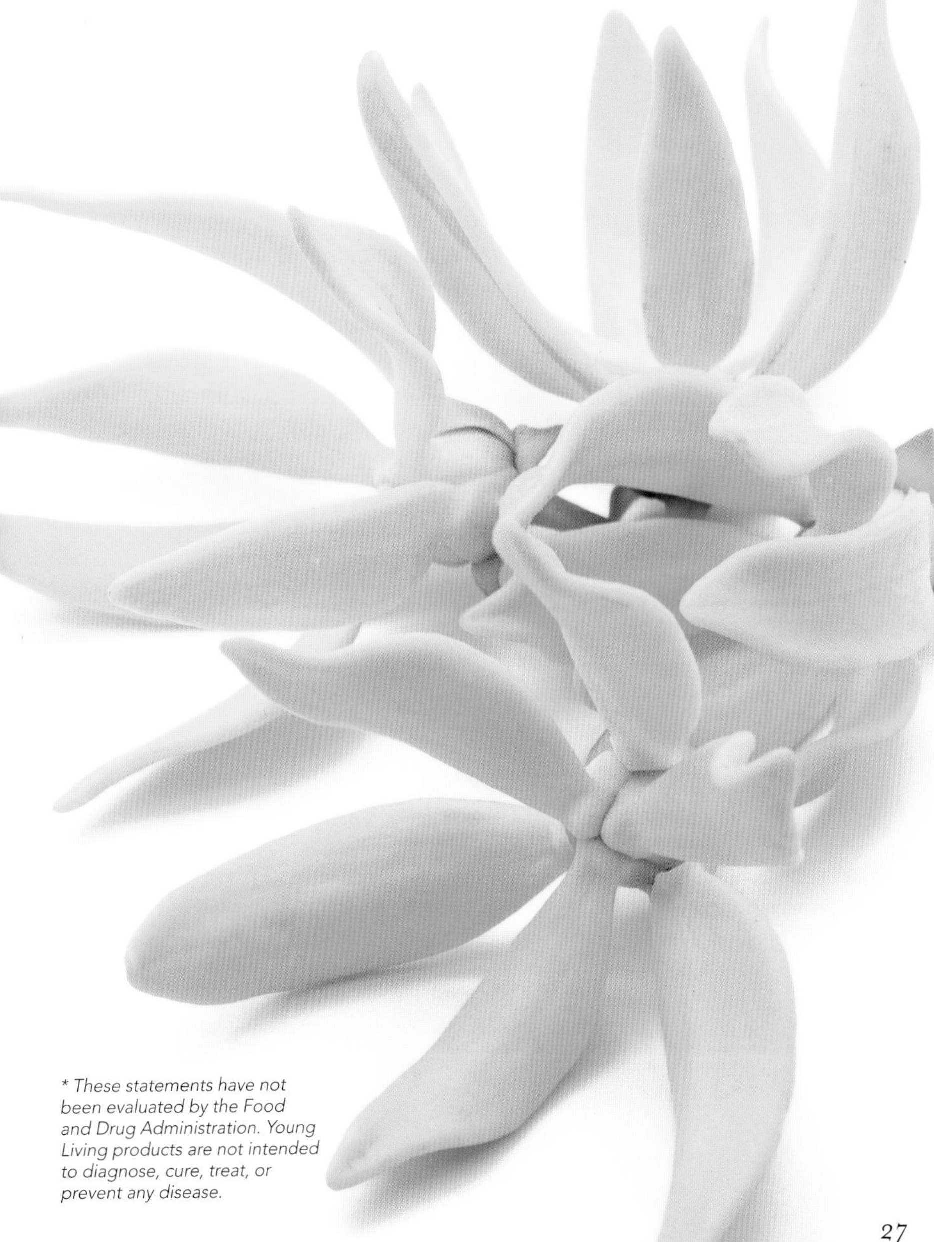

** These statements have not been evaluated by the Food and Drug Administration. Young Living products are not intended to diagnose, cure, treat, or prevent any disease.*

LAVENDER

Aromatic · Tropical

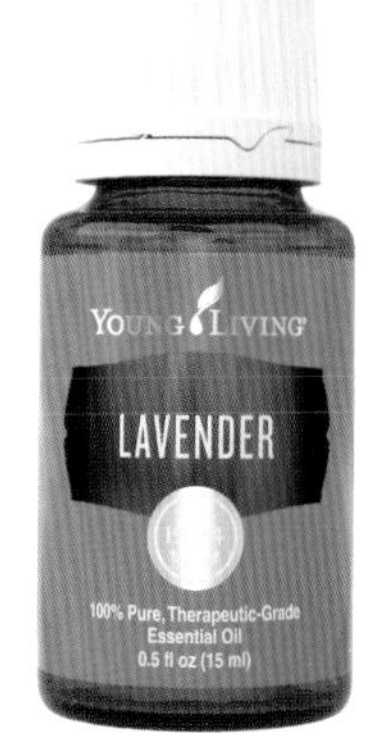

NATURAL CONSTITUENTS

Linalyl Acetate, Linalool, Cis-Beta-Ocimene, Trans-Beta-Ocimene, Terpinen-4-ol

ORAC: 360 µTE/100g

Lavender (lavandula angustifolia) is the most versatile of all essential oils. Therapeutic-grade lavender has been highly regarded for the skin. Lavender has been clinically evaluated for its potential relaxing effects. Historically it was used to cleanse, calm, and promote skin wellness. The fragrance is calming, relaxing and balancing—physically and emotionally. This plant is grown and distilled at Young Living Farms.

This popular oil has long been revered for its calming, soothing fragrance. It's a key ingredient in many calming blends. Diffuse it before bedtime as part of your nighttime routine. It adds the perfect atmosphere for a restful night's sleep and makes the perfect addition to bath, hair, body, and skin care products.

BEST RESULTS

- Known for its comforting and calming aroma.
- Unwind by adding a few drops to a bath.
- Aroma is perfect for diffusing indoors and outdoors to dispel odors.
- Makes a perfect addition to shampoos, lotions, and skin care products.
- A key ingredient in many blends.

BEST RESULTS

- Unwind: enhance your bath with 10 drops in 1 tablespoon of carrier oil. Add to Epsom salts and enjoy.
- Foot massage: gently rub 1-2 drops all over the feet.
- Quiet your thoughts: enjoy a more tranquil spirit by inhaling deeply directly from the bottle.
- Help skin stay smooth: add 10 drops to 1 tablespoon of carrier oil. Use as a daily moisturizer.
- Power down: diffuse for 20 minutes before bedtime as part of your routine before sleep.
- Sparkling nails: add 2 drops to 1 teaspoon of coconut oil and massage into nails and nail beds for calming and smoothing effects.
- Stretch and relax: massage 2-4 drops into your muscles. Stretch and breathe deeply, focusing on letting go of the stress in your day.
- Water fountains: place a drop in your fountain to scent the air, and prolong the time between cleaning.
- Deodorant: rub 2-4 drops over armpit area to act as a deodorant.
- Dry lips: add a drop to a pinch of coconut oil and rub on dry lips.
- Scalp conditioner: rub several drops into the scalp to condition and moisturize.
- Conditioner: rub several drops into the ends of dry or brittle hair.
- Keep it fresh: place a few drops on a cotton ball and place in a linen closet to scent linens.
- Pests: place a few drops on a cotton ball and place in a linen closet to keep pests at bay.
- Create serenity: place a drop on each of the temples, (being careful not to touch the eyes with essential oil) every two hours to re-focus and clear your mind.

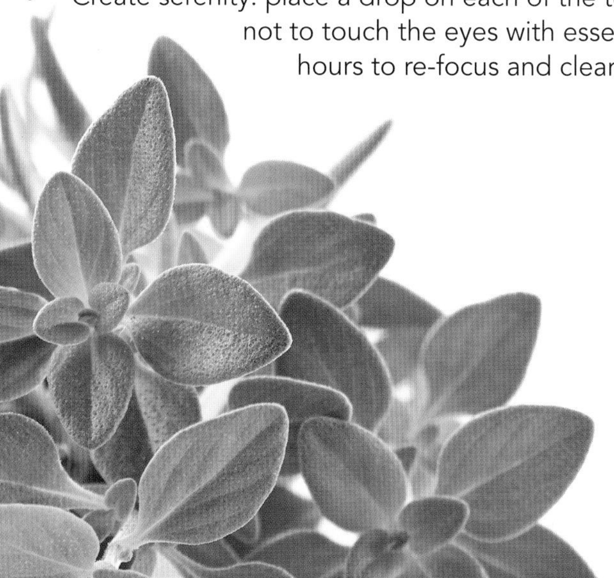

** These statements have not been evaluated by the Food and Drug Administration. Young Living products are not intended to diagnose, cure, treat, or prevent any disease.*

LEMON

Aromatic · Topical

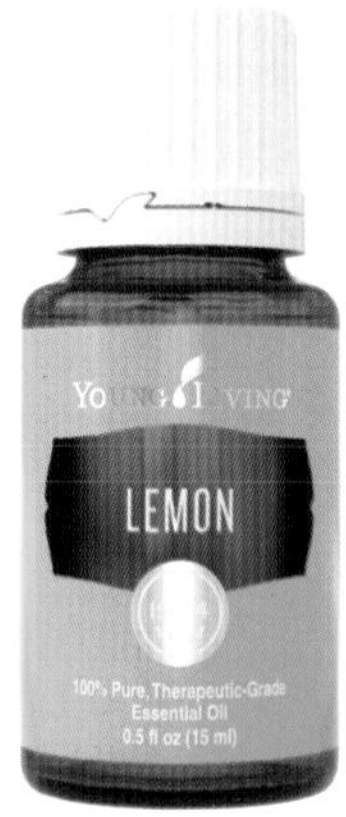

NATURAL CONSTITUENTS

Limonene, Gamma-Terpinene, Beta-Pinene, Alpha-Pinene, Sabinene

Lemon (citrus limon) has been studied for potential antiseptic properties and potential effects on immune function. Caution: citrus oils should not be applied to skin that will be exposed to direct sunlight or ultraviolet light within 72 hours.

BEST RESULTS

- Air freshener: add 6 drops to 6 drops of Purification in a squirt bottle mixed with distilled water to use in bathroom as an air freshener.
- Gum: use 1-2 drops to remove gum.
- Oil: use 1-2 drops to remove oil.
- Grease spots: use 1-2 drops to break up grease spots.
- Crayons: use 1-2 drops to remove crayon.
- Keep fruit fresh: fill a bowl with cool water and add 2-3 drops of Lemon; soak cleaned fruit into the water and stir; be sure all surfaces of the fruit are in contact with the Lemon. Drain, rinse, dry, and place in a bowl.
- Wash the peel: add 2-3 drops to a bowl filled with cool water; drop cleaned fruit into the water and stir; be sure all surfaces of the fruit contact the Lemon. Use a fresh dishcloth to massage the peel. Drain, rinse, and enjoy.
- Freshen the taste: when your fruit starts to smell like stale refrigerator smells, brighten it up by using the same method as above.
- Freshen counter tops: add 2-3 drops to water and spray counters to spruce them up.
- Freshen dishcloths: before dishcloths start to sour, soak them overnight in a bowl of water with 5 drops of Lemon.
- Freshen hands: after using the restroom, wash your hands and rub a drop of Lemon on them.
- Brighten and freshen the house: add 1-2 drops to cotton balls and place in heating/cooling vents.

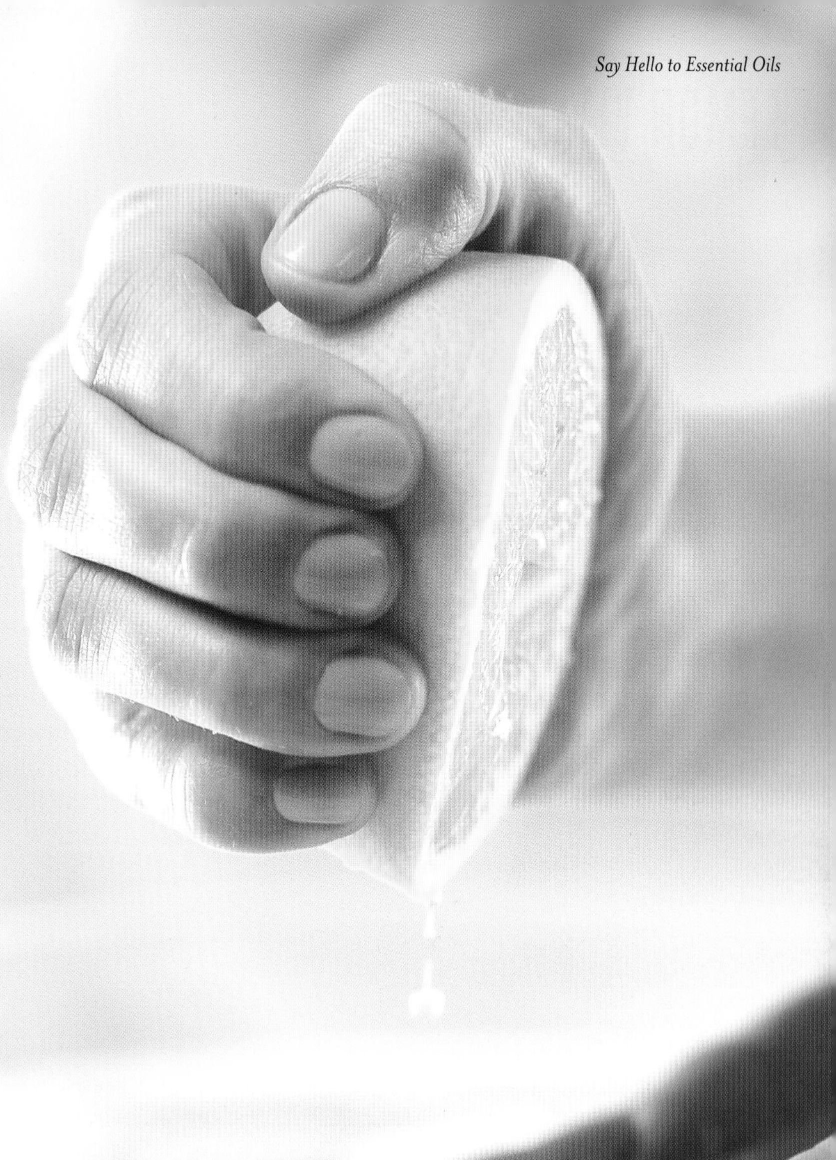

* These statements have not been evaluated by the Food and Drug Administration. Young Living products are not intended to diagnose, cure, treat, or prevent any disease.

LEMON VITALITY™

Dietary Supplement

NATURAL CONSTITUENTS

Limonene, Gamma-Terpinene, Beta-Pinene, Alpha-Pinene, Sabinene

ORAC: 660 μTE/100g

Lemon is considered the most identifiable scent and flavor on earth. This dietary version is an easy way to have the power of fresh lemon zest in your kitchen at all times. The fresh sparkling flavor of Lemon Vitality™ makes it the perfect flavor enhancer for all of your recipes.

Probably one of the most versatile essential oils, Lemon Vitality adds piquant sweetness to everything it touches. It freshens and blends with foods and flavors so seamlessly that no kitchen should be without it. The naturally occurring constituent limonene, revered for its cleansing properties makes Lemon Vitality a great addition to a healthy lifestyle.

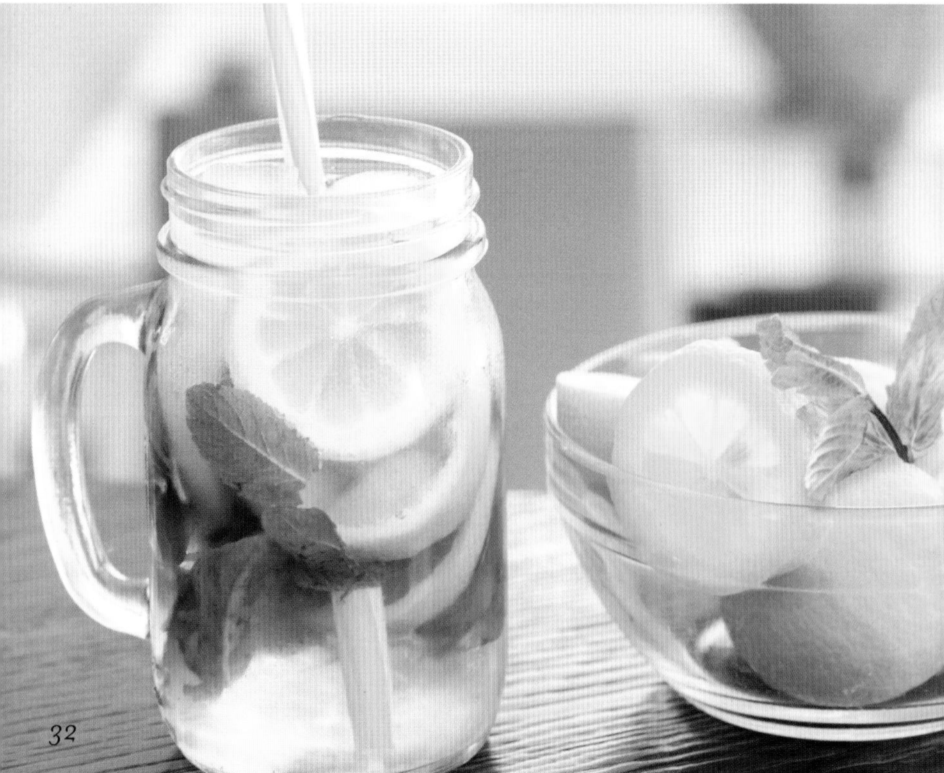

BEST RESULTS

- Lemonade: mix 2 drops with 2 tablespoons of honey and 2 cups of pure water; sweeten to suit your own taste.
- Smoothie: add 2 drops to 1 cup of strawberries, ½ cup of water and 1 tablespoon organic agave syrup. Blend and serve.
- Lemon glaze: add 4 drops to 2 tablespoons of coconut oil. Combine with 2 tablespoons of organic agave syrup and a pinch of sea salt. Whip gently and drizzle on your favorite foods.
- Flavored cream cheese: add 5 drops to 8 ounces of cream cheese and 1 tablespoon of organic agave syrup. Mix well and chill. Use as a fruit dip or a spread for bagels, toast or desserts.
- Hot tonic: add 2 drops to 8 ounces of hot water. Stir in 1 tablespoon of organic agave syrup. Mix well and drink.
- Fish freshening: add 1-2 drops to 1 teaspoon of vinegar and 1 ounce of water in a small food-safe spray bottle. Shake vigorously and spray fish.
- Hollandaise: use 2 drops instead of lemon juice when preparing 4 servings of Hollandaise.
- Salad dressing: add 4 drops to 2 tablespoons of vinegar, 4 tablespoons of water, 1 teaspoon of Worcestershire sauce, and 1 tablespoon of organic agave syrup. Mix well and drizzle over salad.

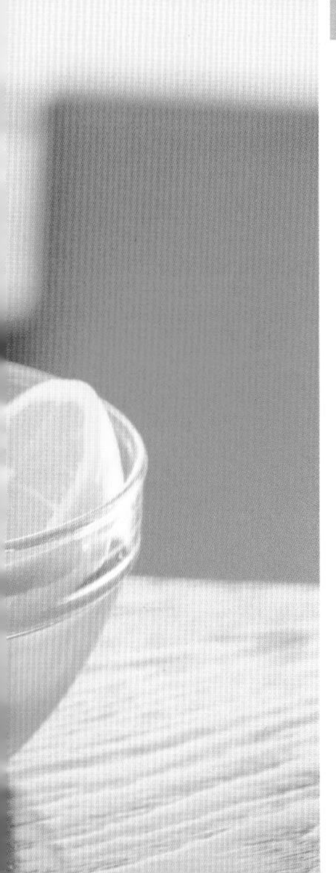

BEST USES

- Revered for its dynamic use in sweet and savory dishes.
- Celebrated for its flavor and freshening aroma.
- Includes the naturally occurring constituent limonene.
- A key ingredient in many health products and essential oil blends.

** These statements have not been evaluated by the Food and Drug Administration. Young Living products are not intended to diagnose, cure, treat, or prevent any disease.*

PANAWAY®

Aromatic · Topical

Contains:
Wintergreen
Helichrysum
Clove
Peppermint

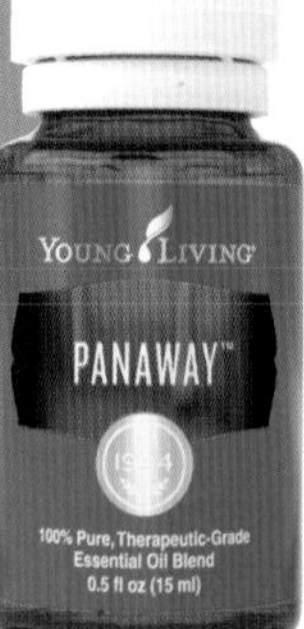

NATURAL CONSTITUENTS

Methyl Salicylate Eugenol, Eugenol Acetate, Beta-Carophyllene Menthol, Menthone, Menthofuran, Eucalpytol, Isomenthone, Neomenthol, Pulegone, Menthyl Acetate

PanAway® is a relief blend of Wintergreen, Clove, Peppermint, and Helichrysum. This blend is meant to support an active lifestyle by providing a warming effect on the skin after activity. This original combination of Wintergreen, Helichrysum, Clove, and Peppermint essential oils is ideal for post-exercise application. The methyl salicylate, gamma-curcumene, menthol, and eugenol are all highly regarded for their cooling, stimulating sensations to the skin.

BEST USES

- Diffuse for a cleansing and refreshing atmosphere.
- Daub 1-3 drops to wrists, chest, base of neck, or bottoms of feet to experience a stimulating and rejuvenating aromatic sensation.
- Combine 1-5 drops with V-6™ Vegetable Oil Complex and massage muscles after exercise.
- Combine 1-2 drops with your favorite moisturizer to complement healthy-looking skin.

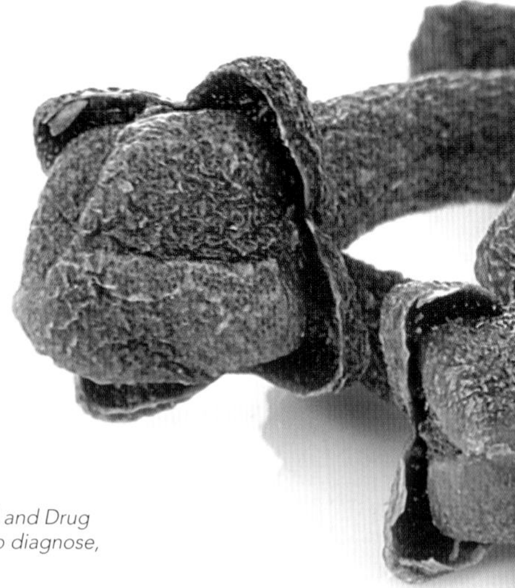

** These statements have not been evaluated by the Food and Drug Administration. Young Living products are not intended to diagnose, cure, treat, or prevent any disease.*

BEST RESULTS

- Stimulating aroma: apply 1-2 drops topically to wrists and décolleté.
- Support healthy skin: apply 1-2 drops topically to appropriate area(s).
- Uplift: rub a drop on the temples, forehead and back of the neck.
- Refreshing body massage: mix with massage oil.
- Cold morning fingers: rub 1-2 drops on fingers and hands to warm and loosen.
- Refreshing back rub: rub 2-3 drops at the base of the spine.
- Refreshing pets: massage 1-2 drops diluted with V-6 vegetable oil on muscles and joints.
- Ease the spirit: diffuse for 1 hour, twice a day.
- Emotional uplift: diffuse for 1 hour, twice a day.
- Warming the back: apply 1-2 drops topically to muscles and along the spine.
- Warming the joints: apply 1-2 drops topically to joint area(s).
- Stimulating foot massage: apply 1-2 drops topically to feet and gently massage.
- Warming the neck: apply 1-2 drops topically to neck.
- Warming abdominal skin: apply topically to abdomen.
- Afternoon lull: apply 1-2 drops topically to scalp, temples, and back of neck.
- Invigorating bath: mix with YL Bath Gel Base in warm water for an invigorating bath.

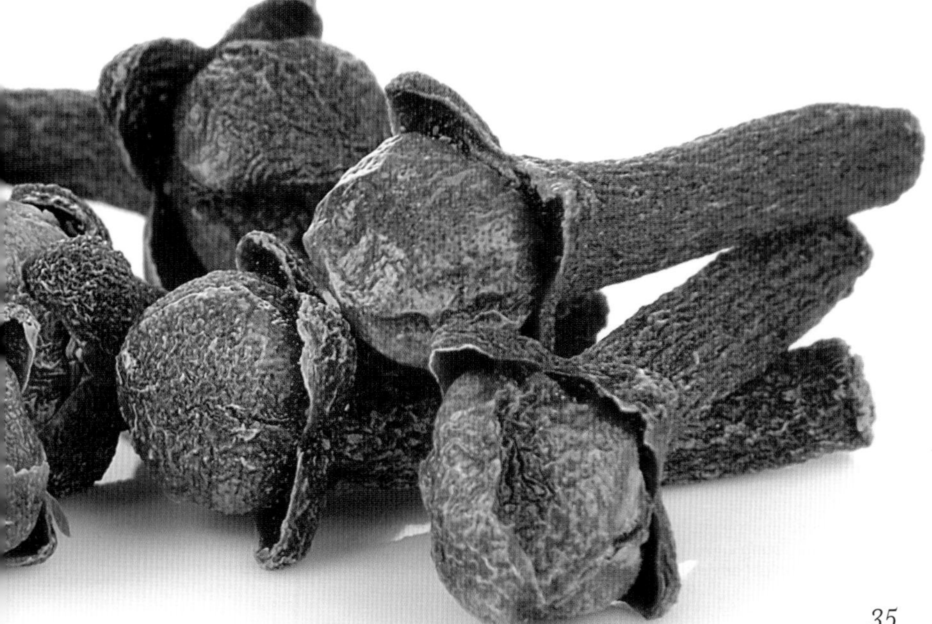

PEPPERMINT

Aromatic · Topical

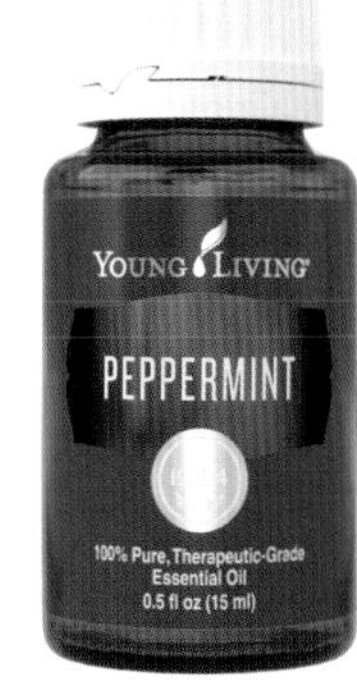

NATURAL CONSTITUENTS

Menthol, Menthone, Menthofuran, Eucalpytol, Isomenthone, Neomenthol, Pulegone, Menthyl Acetate

Peppermint (mentha piperita) is one of the oldest and most highly regarded herbs for soothing digestion. Scientists have researched its effects on the liver and respiratory systems. It has been known for centuries to improve concentration and mental accuracy.

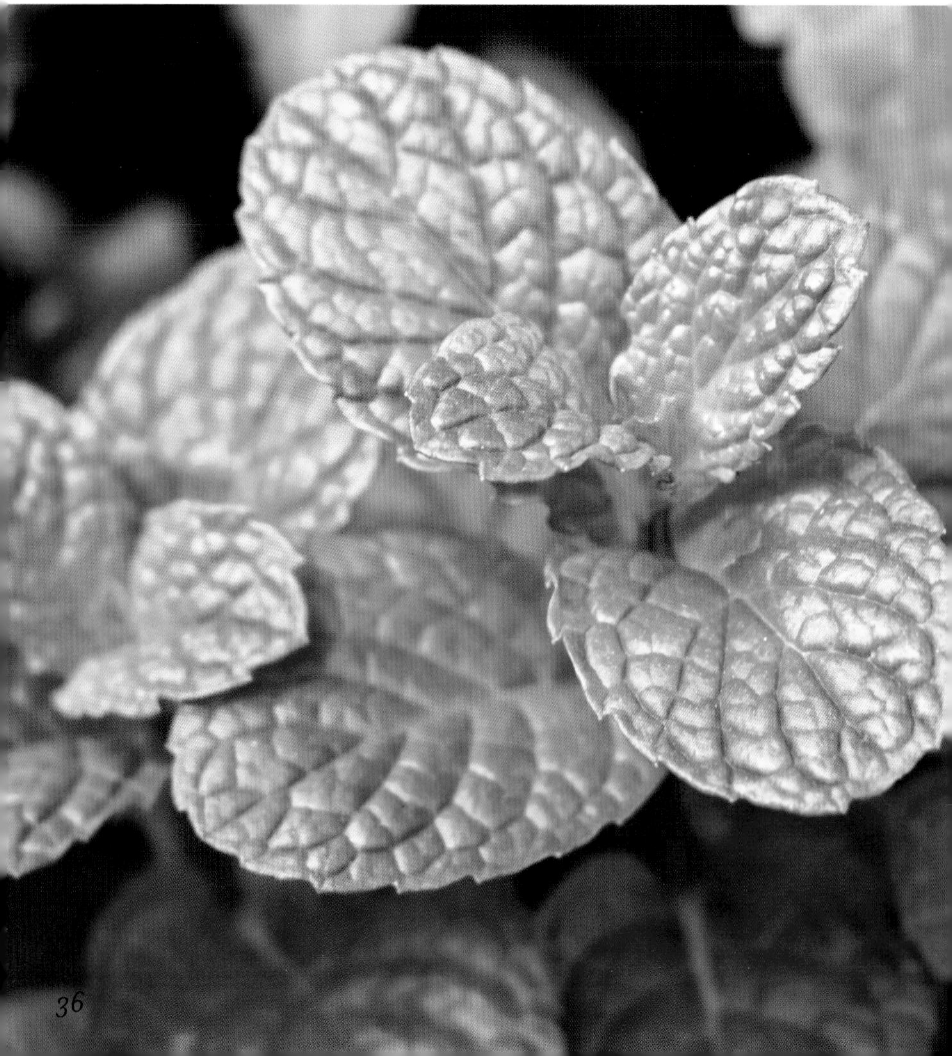

BEST RESULTS

- Working out: diffuse before and during a workout to boost your mood and drive.
- Cooling down: massage on muscles during cool-down for a cool, tingling sensation on the skin.
- Feeling hot: rub several drops on the bottoms of the feet.
- A little pick-me-up: massage several drops on the abdomen.
- Scalp revitalizer: add 1-2 drops to your morning shampoo to give your morning cleansing routine a little boost.
- Afternoon slump: rub a drop on the temples or scalp (stay away from the eyes) and on the back of the neck.
- Support concentration/study: diffuse in the room while studying to improve concentration and accuracy.
- Help with recall: place one drop on the tongue and rub another drop under the nose to improve alertness, concentration, and recall.
- Pests (kitchen): place 2 drops on a cotton ball and place along the path or point of entry.
- Paint fumes: mix a full 15 ml bottle into a 5-gallon can of paint to help dispel the fumes.
- Plant health: add 4-5 drops to 4 ounces of water and spray plants to help repel pests.
- Brighten and freshen the house: add 1-2 drops to cotton balls and place in heating/cooling vents.

BEST USES

- Put 2-3 drops on the floor of your shower for an invigorating aroma and cooling foot effect.
- Following your workout, put 1-2 drops on your neck, temples, and calves for a cooling effect.
- Add 1-2 drops to your bath with Epsom salts for a refreshing soak.

** These statements have not been evaluated by the Food and Drug Administration. Young Living products are not intended to diagnose, cure, treat, or prevent any disease.*

PEPPERMINT VITALITY™

Dietary Supplement

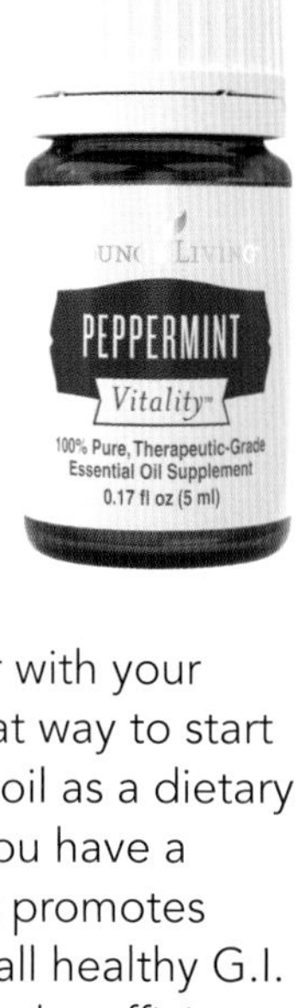

NATURAL CONSTITUENTS

Menthol, Menthone, Menthofuran, Eucalpytol, Isomenthone, Neomenthol, Pulegone, Menthyl Acetate

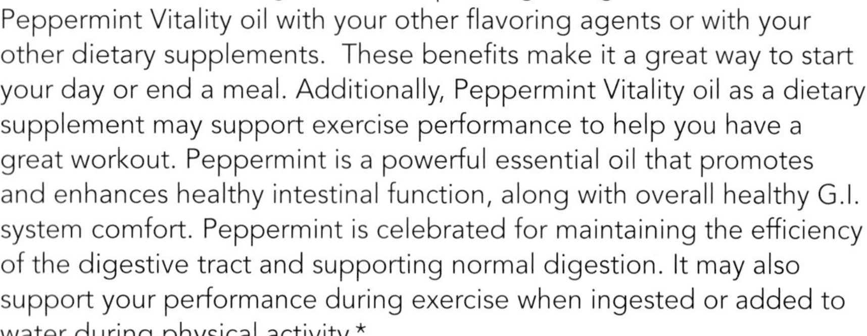

Enjoy the bright, cool flavor of Peppermint Vitality™ essential oil. Not only is the taste stimulating and refreshing, but it also can support gastrointestinal comfort and normal digestion.* Keep Young Living's Peppermint Vitality oil with your other flavoring agents or with your other dietary supplements. These benefits make it a great way to start your day or end a meal. Additionally, Peppermint Vitality oil as a dietary supplement may support exercise performance to help you have a great workout. Peppermint is a powerful essential oil that promotes and enhances healthy intestinal function, along with overall healthy G.I. system comfort. Peppermint is celebrated for maintaining the efficiency of the digestive tract and supporting normal digestion. It may also support your performance during exercise when ingested or added to water during physical activity.*

BEST USES

- Add 1-2 drops to impart foods and beverages with an airy, crisp freshness.
- Add to recipes to support gastrointestinal system comfort,* promote healthy bowel function,* enhance healthy gut function,* maintain efficiency of the digestive tract,* and support normal digestion.*
- Put 1-2 drops in water to support performance during exercise.*

** These statements have not been evaluated by the Food and Drug Administration. Young Living products are not intended to diagnose, cure, treat, or prevent any disease.*

BEST RESULTS

- Minty refresh: add a drop to herbal tea.
- Working out: diffuse before and during a workout to boost your mood and drive.
- Summer cooler: drink a drop mixed in a glass of cold water to cool off on a hot day.
- Mint lemonade: add 1-2 drops to 8 ounces of lemonade for a summertime favorite.
- Peppermint glaze: add 4 drops to 2 tablespoons of coconut oil. Combine with 2 tablespoons of organic agave syrup and a pinch of sea salt. Whip gently and drizzle on your favorite foods.
- Workout: add 1-2 drops to your hydration water during your workout for a refreshing, bold taste.
- Indigestion: add 1-2 drops to 4 ounces of water. Stir and drink quickly.
- Reducing coffee intake: place a drop in a cup of hot water and enjoy in place of coffee.
- Coffee enhancement: place a drop in coffee to give it bright flavor and zing.
- Flavoring: add 2 drops to recipes in place of extract.
- Preservative: add to food as a preservative.

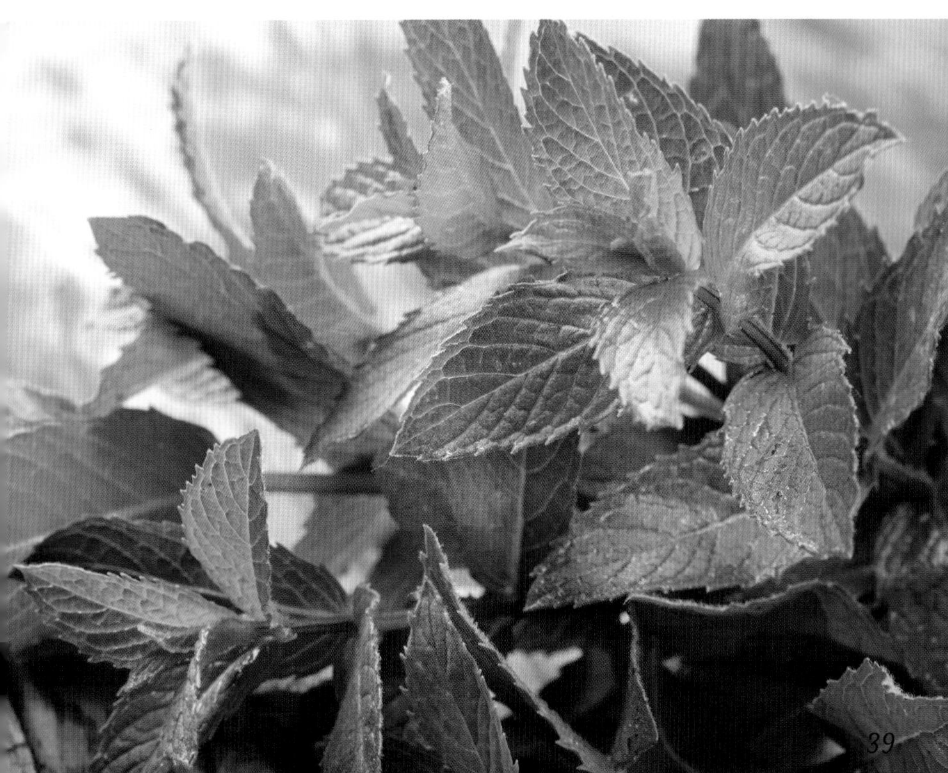

PURIFICATION

Aromatic · Topical

Contains:
Citronella
Rosemary
Lemongrass
Melaleuca Alternifolia
Lavandin
Myrtle

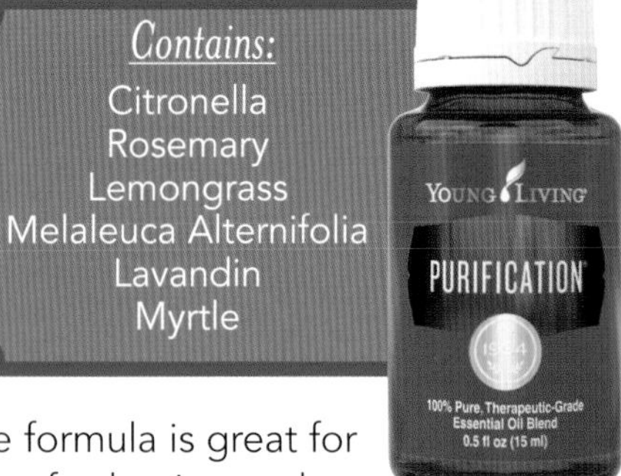

NATURAL CONSTITUENTS

Cineol, Neral (Citral B), and Geranial (Citral A)

Purification® is blend of Citronella, Lemongrass, Rosemary, Melaleuca, Lavandin and Myrtle. The formula is great for diffusing—particularly for brightening, freshening and refining the air and neutralizing mildew, cigarette smoke, and disagreeable odors. The essential oil profile in this blend is perfect for freshening even the most persistent odors—inside and outside. The unique combination combines the powerful naturally occurring compounds cineol, neral, and geranial—all of them acclaimed for their aromatic properties. Add Purification oil to moisturizers to improve the appearance of healthy-looking skin or apply topically to enjoy the outdoors annoyance-free.

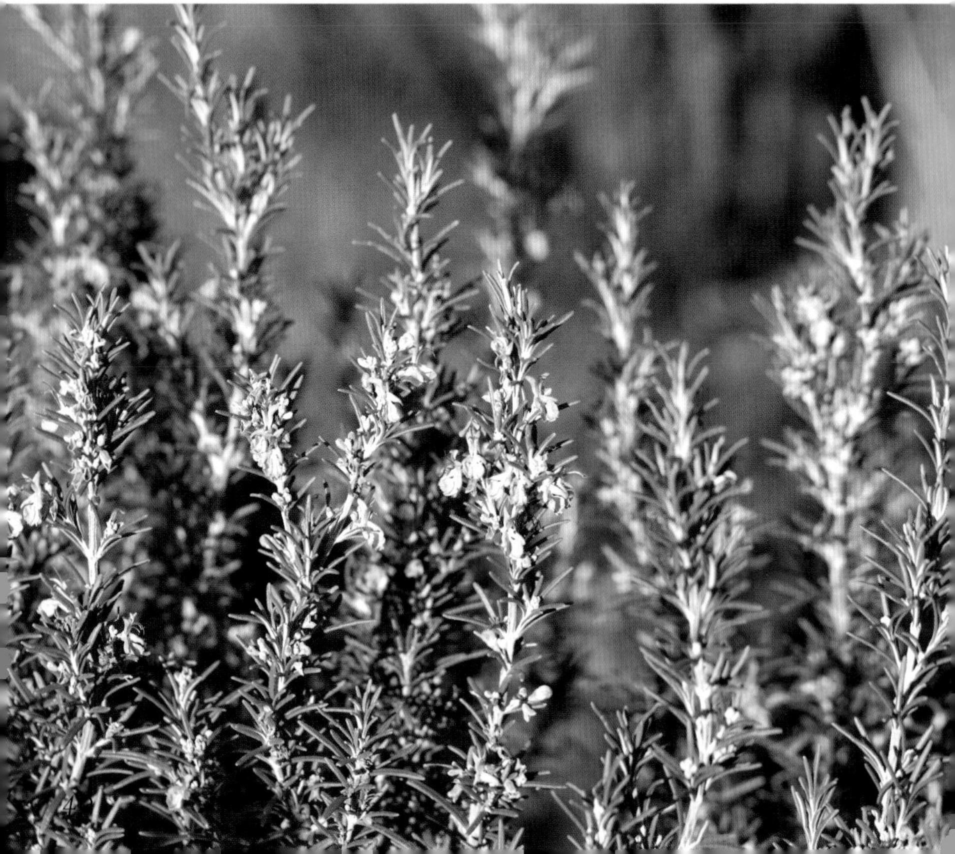

BEST USES

- Combine 1-5 drops with V-6™ Vegetable Oil Complex and massage feet for a soothing and relaxing experience.
- Diffuse indoors and outdoors to dispel odors.
- Add 1-2 drops to cotton balls and place in air vents to revitalize the air.
- Add to your favorite bath or shower base.
- Add 4 drops to a cup of Epsom salts for a soothing bath.
- Add to distilled water in a small spray bottle and use when traveling to freshen air.
- Combine 1-2 drops with your favorite moisturizer to complement healthy-looking skin.
- Apply topically to enjoy the outdoors annoyance-free.

BEST RESULTS

- Air freshener: diffuse to neutralize foul or stale odors.
- Fresh vents: put several drops on a cotton ball and place in the air vents in the home, office, car, hotel room or enclosed areas.
- Fresh travel: while traveling, inhale during flights to give yourself a boost in re-circulated air.
- Sneaker odors: put 2 drops on 2 cotton balls and place in the toes of smelly sneakers to combat odors.
- Humidifier: place a drop on each end of a cotton swab and place on top of your cold water humidifier to brighten and freshen the air.
- Pest free outdoors: spritz several drops mixed with water to enjoy the outdoors annoyance-free.
- Pet earwax: combine with Peppermint and dilute with V6 vegetable oil. Add to cotton swab and rub just inside the pet's ears to eliminate earwax and odor.
- Freshen air: diffuse into the air where moldy, sour, or stuffy smells are present.
- Stimulating bath: mix with YL Bath Gel Base in warm water for a stimulating bath.
- Water fountains: place a drop in your fountain to scent the air, and prolong the time between cleaning.

** These statements have not been evaluated by the Food and Drug Administration. Young Living products are not intended to diagnose, cure, treat, or prevent any disease.*

R.C.™

Aromatic · Topical

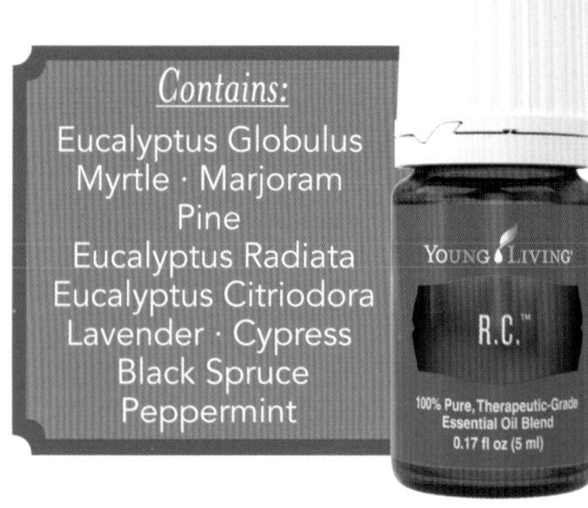

NATURAL CONSTITUENTS

Limonene, Linalool acetate, Linalool, Camphene, Eucalyptol

R.C.™ essential oil blend is a unique combination of Cypress, Spruce, and three types of Eucalyptus (E. globulus, E. radiata, and E citriodora) oils and includes the naturally occurring constituent limonene. Rub R.C. on feet, temples, back of neck, forehead, chakra, and Vita Flex points for an elevating, emboldening aromatic sensation.

BEST USES

- Daub 1-3 drops to wrists, chest, base of neck, or bottoms of feet to experience a stimulating and rejuvenating aromatic sensation.
- Add to V-6™ Vegetable Oil Complex to create a spa-like, soothing atmosphere with massage.
- Rub 1-3 drops on feet or chest before exercising to create an uplifting and inspiring aroma.
- Diffuse to create a comforting aroma.

BEST RESULTS

- Process your negative emotions by directly inhaling the aroma from the bottle.
- Add 1-2 drops to 4-ounce glass spray bottle. Shake well and mist the air to enjoy the aroma.
- When confronting difficult smells or fumes, add 1-2 drops to a teaspoon of coconut oil and brush across the upper lip. The aroma can help you cope with or even overcome the bad odor.

** These statements have not been evaluated by the Food and Drug Administration. Young Living products are not intended to diagnose, cure, treat, or prevent any disease.*

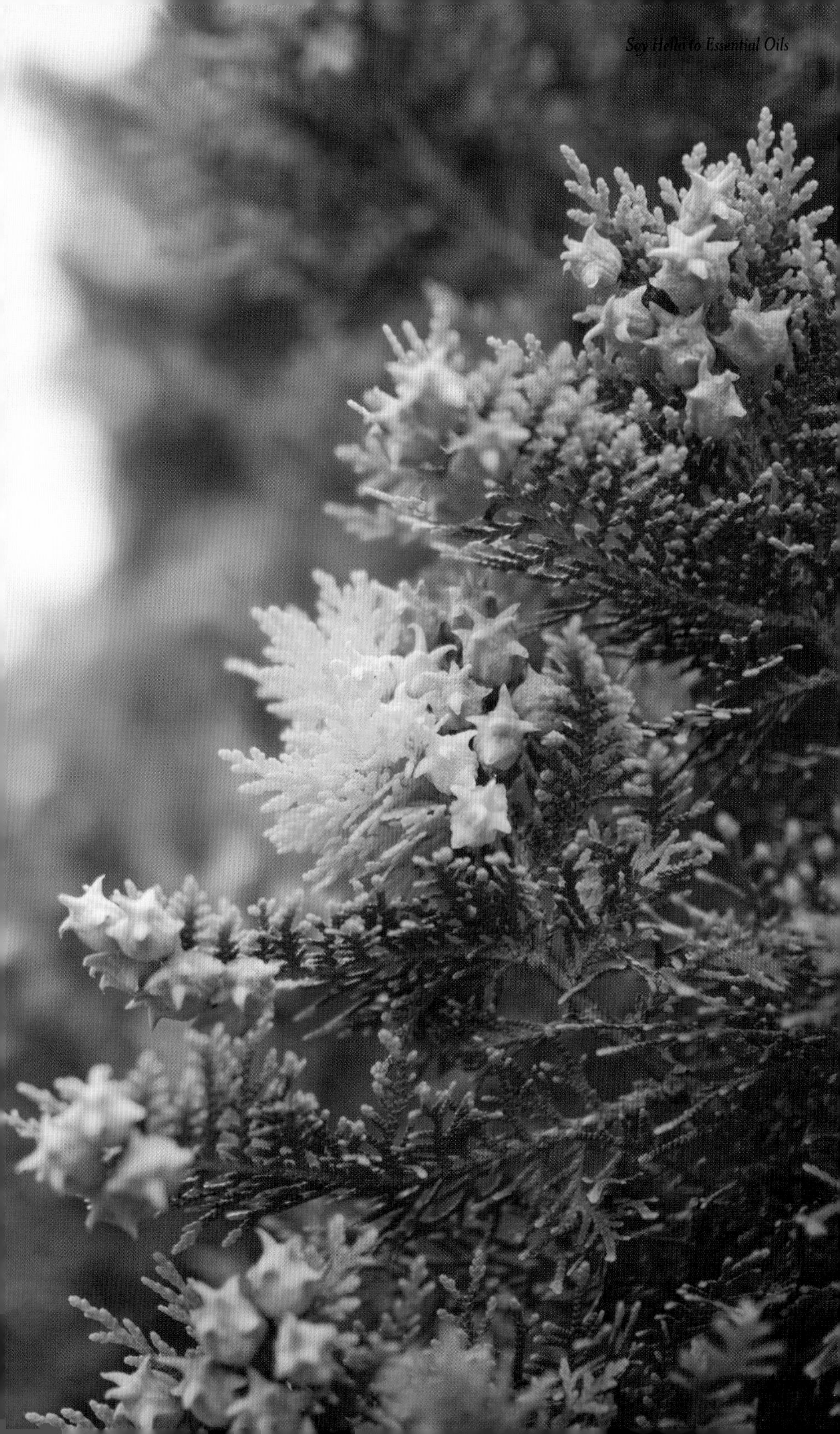

STRESS AWAY™

Aromatic · Topical

Contains:
Copaiba
Lime
Cedarwood
Vanilla
Ocotea
Lavender

NATURAL CONSTITUENTS

Beta-caryophyllene, Alpha-humulene, Limonene, Cedrol, Eugenol, and Linalool

Stress Away™ is a calming blend of Copaiba, Lime, Cedarwood, Vanilla, Ocotea and Lavender. Stress Away is a unique reformulated essential oil blend designed to help you unwind as you face the hassles, worries, and agitations that creep into everyday life. Stress Away is a unique blend that combines the emotional relaxation* benefits of lime and vanilla. Stress Away also includes Copaiba and Lavender to open the mind and restore emotional balance. Featuring powerful plant constituents, such as the cedrol found in cedarwood and the eugenol that occurs naturally in vanilla, Stress Away can help support a relaxing atmosphere and create an emotionally safe space of comfort, stability, and serenity.

BEST USES

- Diffuse for a mildly sharp aroma with sweet and zesty tones.
- Daub 1-3 drops to wrists, chest, base of neck, or bottoms of feet to experience a stimulating and rejuvenating aromatic sensation.
- Combine 1-5 drops with V-6™ Vegetable Oil Complex and massage muscles after exercise.
- Add 1-2 drops to cotton balls and place in air vents to revitalize the air.

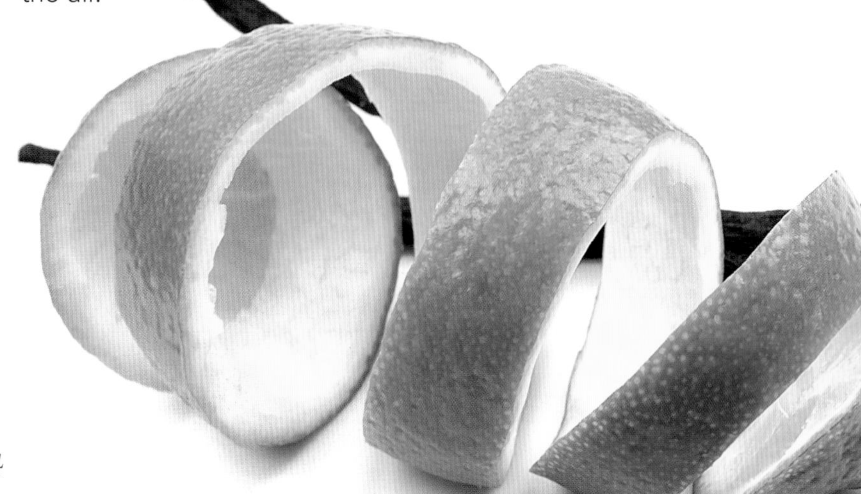

BEST RESULTS

- Increase your calm feeling by rubbing 1-2 drops on the back of the neck, temples, chest, shoulders, wrist, and/or back.
- Soothe yourself by diffusing in half-hour increments.
- Increase your emotional balance by applying generously to the neck, temples, and chest.
- Boost your compassion! Apply generously to the neck, temples, and chest to improve feelings of sensitivity and compassion.
- Promote relaxation in your home and office; diffuse into the air or inhale directly from the bottle.
- Enjoy a relaxing massage by adding 1-2 drops to massage oil to unwind and enjoy a peaceful massage.
- Create an evening ritual - diffuse into the air or dilute 2-5 drops into 1 ounce of water and gently mist the air or linens.
- Relax with a tranquil bath. Mix a few oils of your choice in a 1/2 cup of Epsom salts or YL Bath Gel Base and dissolve in warm bath water for the perfect, tranquil experience.
- Dilute as necessary and apply topically to the back, bottoms of the feet, or back of the neck.
- Clear your mind and apply on hands, cup over nose and mouth, and inhale deeply or diffuse.
- Prepare children for bed: diffuse into the air or dilute 2-5 drops into 1 ounce of water and gently mist the air.
- Diffuse while sleeping.
- Combat the day when you wear it as a perfume by applying 1-2 drops to each wrist and 1 drop to décolleté.
- Relax your feet by rubbing several drops on the bottoms of the feet and massage gently.
- Alleviate frustration by rubbing a drop of oil over the heart and on the bottom of each foot.

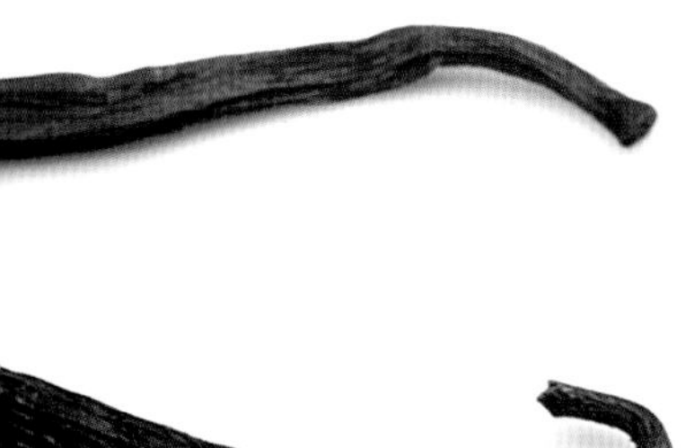

** These statements have not been evaluated by the Food and Drug Administration. Young Living products are not intended to diagnose, cure, treat, or prevent any disease.*

TEA TREE (MELALEUCA ALTERNIFOLIA)

Aromatic · Topical

NATURAL CONSTITUENTS

Terpinen-4-ol, Gamma-Terpinene, Alpha-Terpinene, Eucalyptol, Alpha-Terpineol, Para-Cymene, Limonene, Aromadendrene, Delta-Cadinene, Apha-Pinene

Tea Tree (also known as melaleuca alternifolia), has been highly regarded for its healthful properties. It can be found in a wide spectrum of skin care and spa products that can comfort and support the vitality of healthy-looking skin, scalp, and hair. With a fresh, crisp aroma, Tea Tree essential oil is an important oil in many essential oil blends, as well as in topical skin-care products. When applied topically, Tea Tree can help support healthy-looking hair and scalp, reduce the appearance of blemishes, and can be applied to feet and toenails as needed.*

BEST RESULTS

- Daub 1-2 drops onto a cotton swab. Apply to blemishes to help minimize their appearance.
- Massage 1-2 drops directly into the feet to support healthy feet.
- Massage 1-2 directly into the toenails and nail beds to support healthy toenails.
- To support healthy fingernails, massage 1-2 directly into the fingernails and nail beds.
- Explore new ways to enjoy the outdoors! Diffuse or apply 1-2 drops to the neck and wrists while outdoors for an annoyance-free experience.
- Combine one drop with one drop of Lavender, and one drop of Frankincense and apply to scalp for moisture and shine.
- To address dry skin, combine one drop with one drop of Lavender, and one drop of Frankincense and apply to affected areas.
- Diffuse to enhance the air and deodorize.
- Rub a drop on a rough skin spot mornings and evenings to help it stay smooth.
- Uplift your spirits by applying topically to forehead, temples, base of skull and behind the ears and/or diffuse into the air and inhale.

** These statements have not been evaluated by the Food and Drug Administration. Young Living products are not intended to diagnose, cure, treat, or prevent any disease.*

BEST USES

- Complements healthy-looking skin.
- Has a stimulating and invigorating fragrance.
- Aroma is perfect for diffusing indoors and outdoors to dispel odors.
- Daub 1-3 drops to wrists, chest, base of neck, or bottoms of feet to experience a stimulating and rejuvenating aromatic sensation.
- Combine 1-5 drops with V-6™ Vegetable Oil Complex and massage muscles after exercise.
- Add 1-2 drops to cotton balls and place in air vents to revitalize the air.

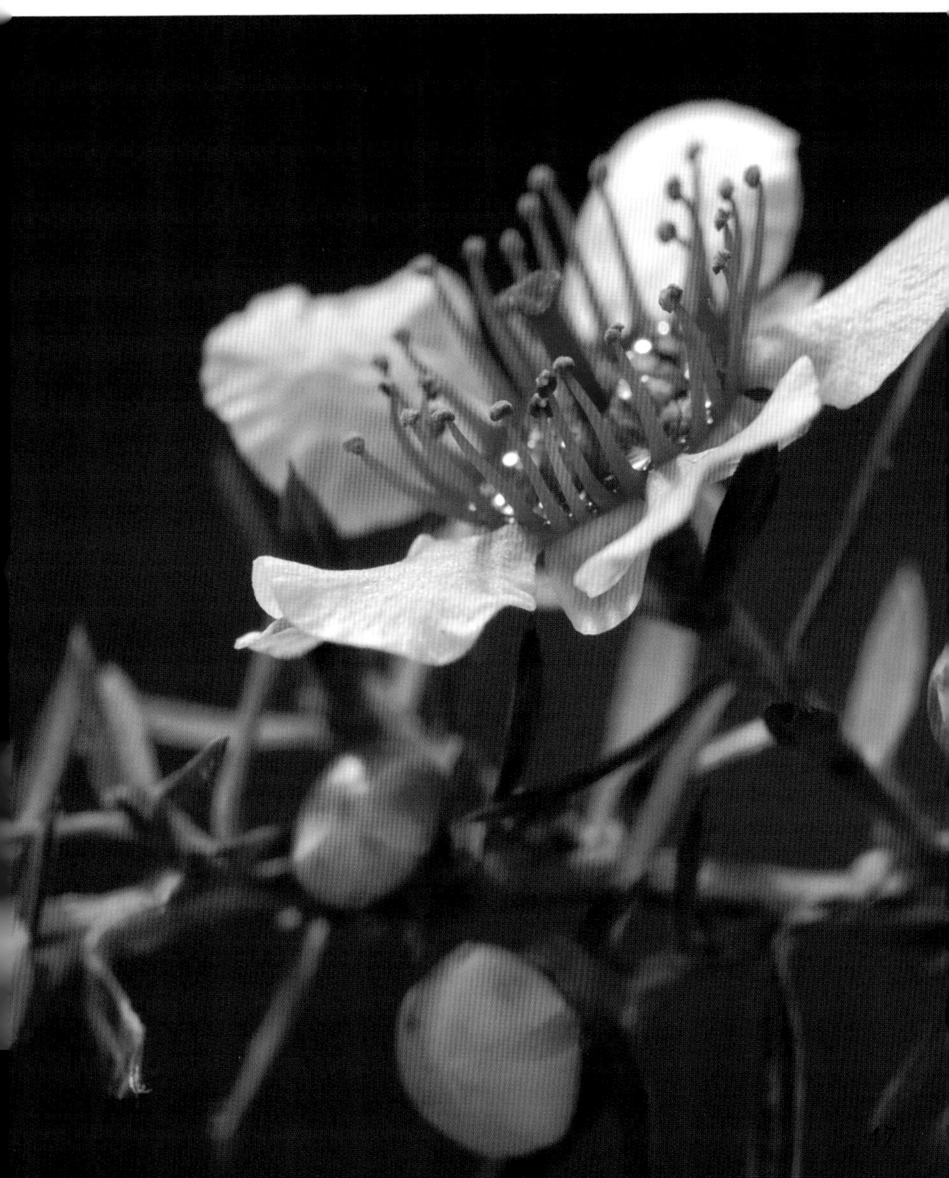

THIEVES®

Aromatic · Topical

Contains:
Clove
Lemon
Cinnamon Bark
Eucalyptus Radiata
Rosemary

NATURAL CONSTITUENTS

Limonene, Eugenol, and Eucalyptol

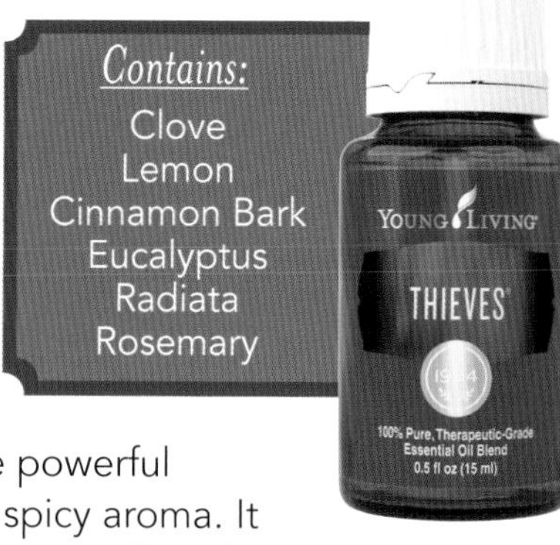

Thieves® is a traditional blend of Clove, Lemon, Cinnamon Bark, Eucalyptus Radiata, and Rosemary. The powerful combination fills any space with a rich, spicy aroma. It is inspired by the legend of four, 15th-century French thieves, who formulated a special aromatic combination while robbing the dead and dying. Thieves is one of Young Living's most popular products. With the benefits of Thieves oil, including cleaning power and an irresistibly spicy scent, Young Living offers it as an essential oil blend and as an important ingredient in a full range of home cleaning and personal care products, from dish soap to toothpaste.

BEST USES

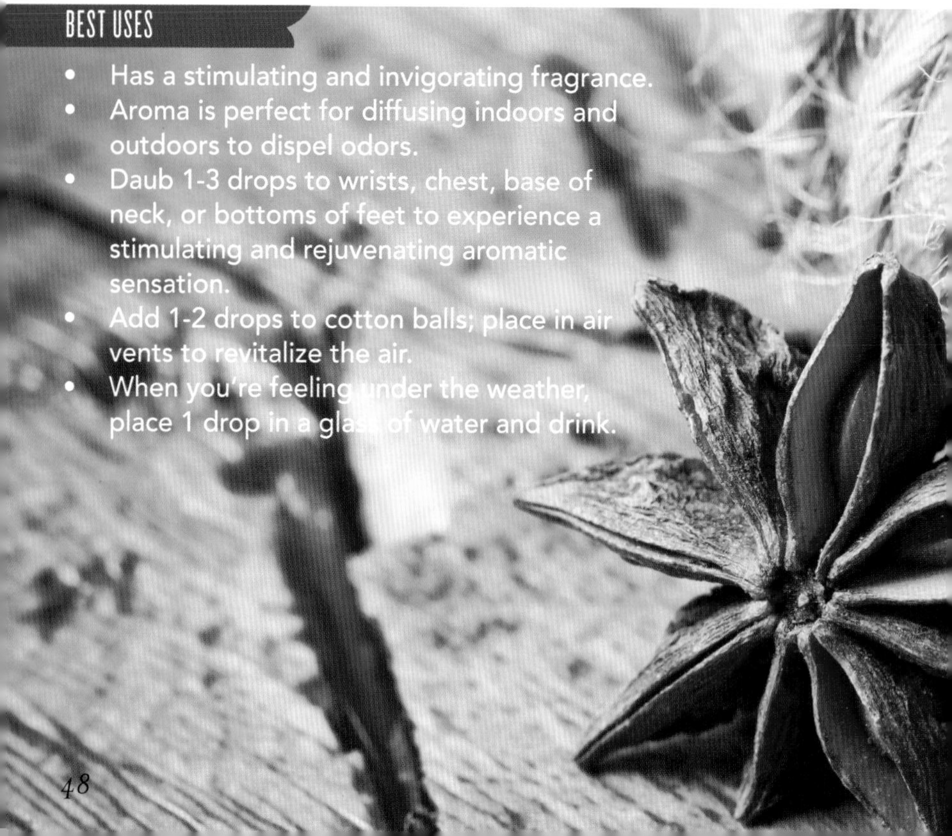

- Has a stimulating and invigorating fragrance.
- Aroma is perfect for diffusing indoors and outdoors to dispel odors.
- Daub 1-3 drops to wrists, chest, base of neck, or bottoms of feet to experience a stimulating and rejuvenating aromatic sensation.
- Add 1-2 drops to cotton balls; place in air vents to revitalize the air.
- When you're feeling under the weather, place 1 drop in a glass of water and drink.

BEST RESULTS

- To create a peaceful environment, diffuse in half-hour increments in each room of the house.
- For sore feet, rub a drop on the bottom of feet. Massage gently.
- Diffuse in half-hour increments to dispel cooking odors while maintaining a warm, inviting atmosphere.
- Refresh your bathroom by diffusing after use.
- Refresh carpets by adding 10 drops to a cup of baking soda. Combine, shake, and sprinkle over carpets before vacuuming.
- Add 10 drops to a cup of baking soda. Mix well and put in shallow bowl in the refrigerator overnight to absorb food odors.
- Dilute 50-50 with V-6 oil and apply to throat and neck; apply a warm compress.
- Keep your house fresh! Place 2-6 drops in a small spray bottle and fill with water; spray countertops, bathtubs, toilets, sinks, and doorknobs.
- Remove the moldy, musty smells; diffuse in half-hour increments in basement and attic to dispel moldy odors.

** These statements have not been evaluated by the Food and Drug Administration. Young Living products are not intended to diagnose, cure, treat, or prevent any disease.*

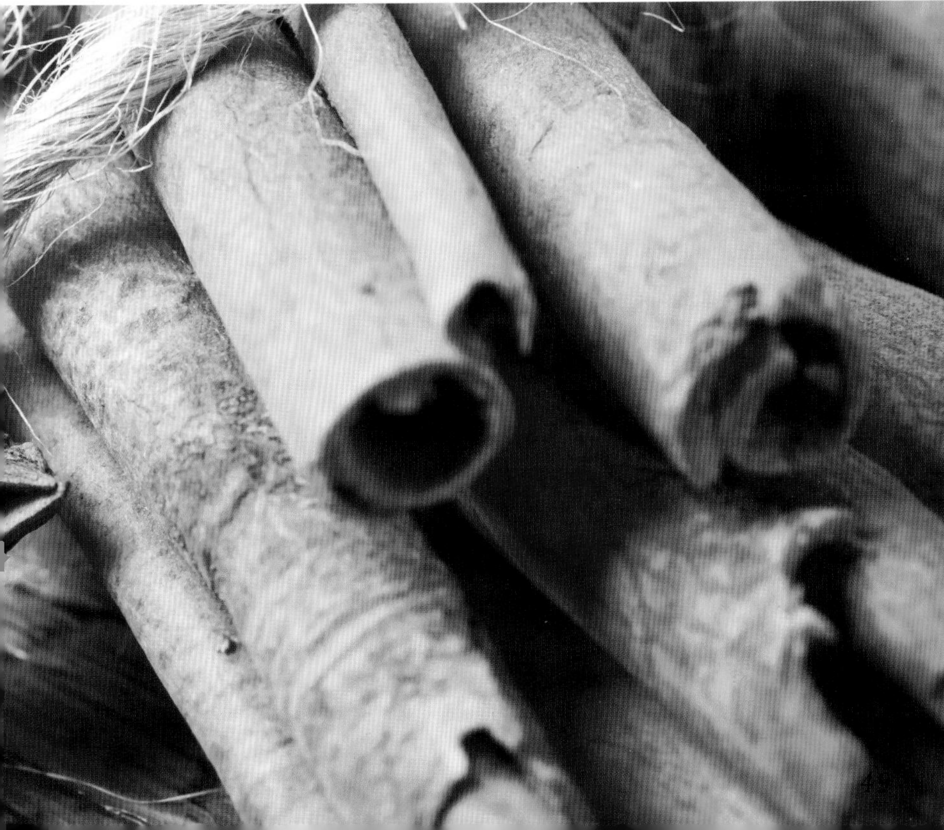

THIEVES® VITALITY™

Dietary Supplement

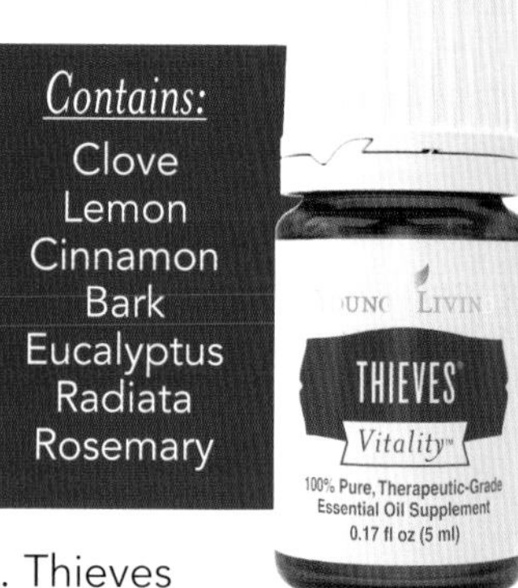

NATURAL CONSTITUENTS

Limonene, Eugenol, and Eucalyptol

Thieves Vitality™ is a powerful blend of Lemon, Clove, Eucalyptus Radiata, Cinnamon Bark, and Rosemary essential oils and is one of our most popular products. Thieves Vitality may help support healthy immune function and contribute to overall wellness when taken as a dietary supplement. These ingredients synergistically combine to offer one of the key benefits of Thieves Vitality oil: overall wellness and support of a healthy immune system. The Eucalyptus Radiata essential oil may help maintain a healthy respiratory system. This blend delivers the naturally derived constituents limonene, eugenol, and eucalyhptol and can be a great addition to food and drinks as a flavoring.*

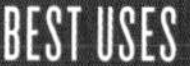

BEST USES

- Add to food or beverages to enhance the flavor. A drop in hot drinks adds a spicy zing.
- May contribute to overall wellness when taken as a dietary supplement.*
- Supports healthy immune function.*
- Add 1 drop Thieves to 2 drops Orange essential oil as a refreshing flavor to complement your favorite beverage.

BEST RESULTS

- When you're feeling under the weather, place 1 drop in a glass of water and drink.
- To freshen your breath, place 2-4 drops in water and gargle as needed.
- Have a scratchy throat? Try diluting 5 drops in 2 tablespoons of vegetable oil. Gargle, spit it out, and rinse with water.
- Support healthy gums by diluting 1 drop in 1 tablespoon of vegetable oil. Using a swab, gently apply to the gums 2 times a day.
- Enjoy a spicy delight by adding a drop to your morning beverage to give it a boost.

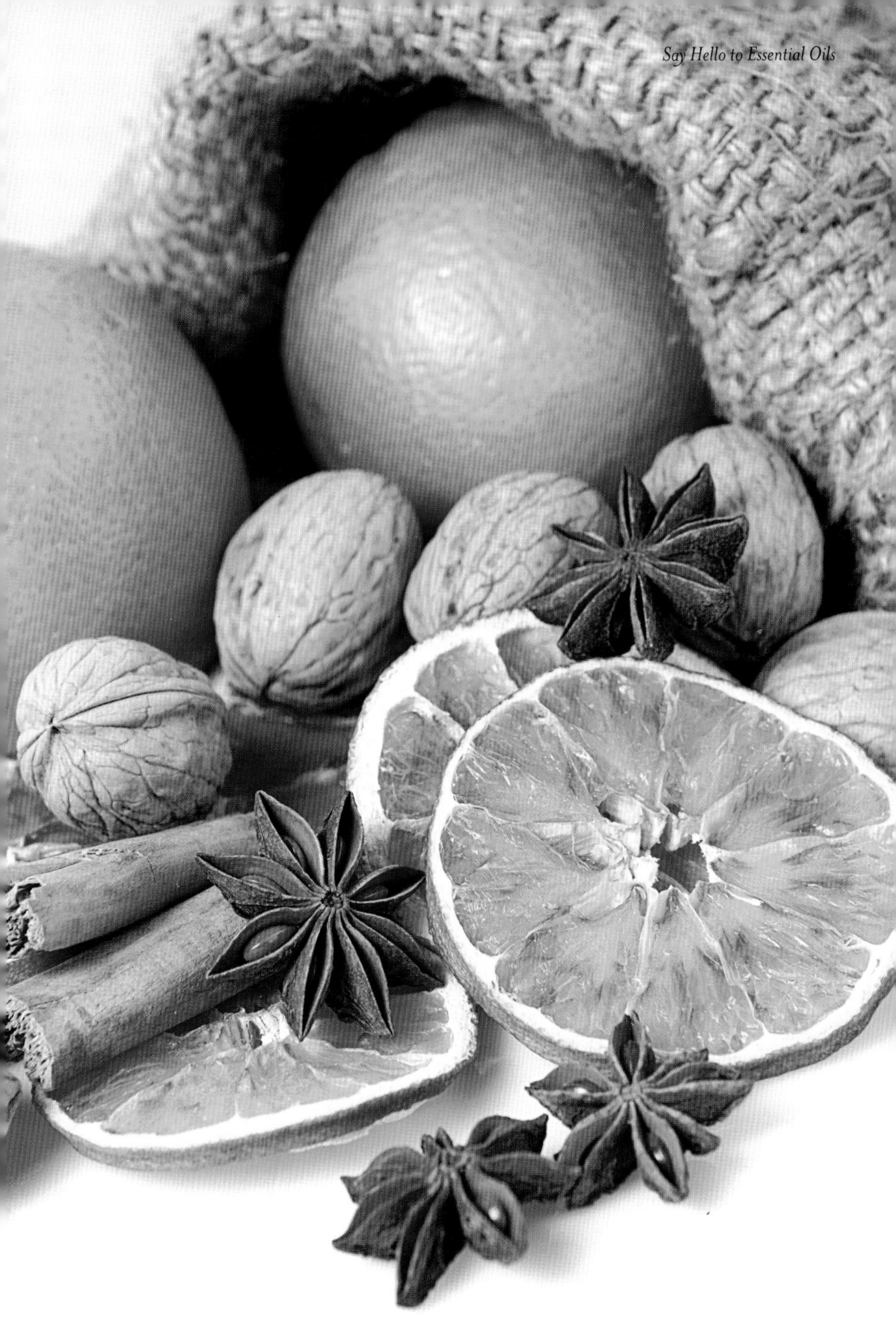

* These statements have not been evaluated by the Food and Drug Administration. Young Living products are not intended to diagnose, cure, treat, or prevent any disease.

THE PATH TO SUCCESS

At first, the dream of advancing to that next rank seems like just that—a dream. But making it a reality is easier than you think. When asked, there are several factors that leaders have said were game-changers for their success.

1) Connect with Leaders

Hands down, the number one thing successful members report is that they had support. No one who has made Silver in Six magically did it alone. Most achievers report that they had strong leaders in their upline. They attribute their success to guiding, coaching, and encouragement. Because most people need guidance in using essential oils, the same holds true for learning how to share. Most members buy their starter kits from people they know and trust and who are available to answer questions.

Leaders with great educational and support tools make all the difference. However, most people don't have a clear source or great access to ideal support. For people who don't have an immediate connection, try searching for like-minded folks on Facebook. Send an invitation to leaders in your upline. Try looking for people who use oils the way you do on social media. Study the people who are doing things the way you see yourself doing them. Ask if they would be willing to add you to their closed Facebook group or start one with them.

2) #1 Way to Sign: Introduction Classes

While make-and-takes are great for customers, it takes a special kind of environment to attract good business builders. People who want to hit the next title quickly learn that they have better leverage for signups when they hold regular classes. This may mean traveling around your county or even to another state. Hitting the road can have huge payoffs with well-planned and well-presented Introduction Classes. Offer to hold these for the distributors that sign up underneath you.

With these events, being consistent is key. Not only that, but creating the ***right*** mix of people in the class makes a HUGE difference. Stack the class with a percentage of positive people who aren't new to the concept. They can help to bring optimism and energy to the rest of the brand-new people. Vicki Opfer covers this really well with her consistently updated Heart-Centered Sharing PDF. Simply enter "heart centered sharing 2015" in a Google search to find and download her free PDF.

Introduction classes become really important when you get to Stacking or Strategic Placement. If you invite your leader into your process, you can use their experience to put the ***right*** members of your team in the right places to be sure your PV is consistent and that it constantly flows upward. Good leaders will be able to help you "get the lights to all turn on," so to speak. This will help you get all of your overrides and bonuses.

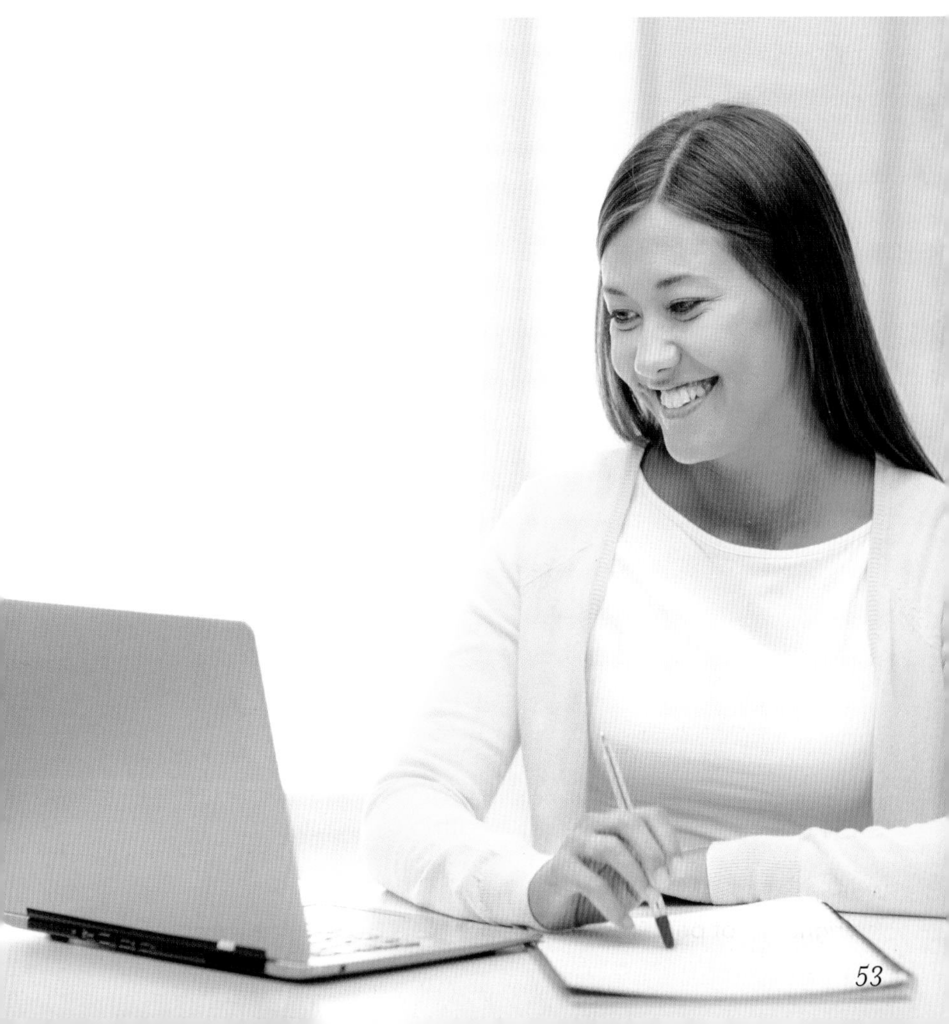

3) Social, Social, Social, Social, Social, Social Media

Why so many different ***socials***? Just as the three most important things in real estate are location, location, location, so too are the top ways to boost your sharing—social media, social media, social media. The brave new world of sharing uses these social media platforms because of their ability to help you leverage time and effort. You'd be surprised how many people will join as members or become business-building distributors on Facebook. Even better, posting your experiences with the oils and how you used them can be a powerful, credibility-building way to share. Many people will ask about a post on Twitter or Instagram, and you can use these to start a great dialogue. YouTube videos can reach an even wider pool of potential team members. Posting pictures with recipes is a great way to promote on Pinterest. Start with posting your love of Young Living products on Facebook, Instagram, and Twitter. Once you have a good group of followers, you might want to create a closed Facebook support group.

Be sure to link all of your social media together to get the best traction. Social media acts as a net. Certain types of people will use different channels. Some people love Pinterest. Some are Twitter addicts. The point is to try and get your message out through as many channels as possible. If you want more fish, you need more boats with nets, right? Think of social media this way.

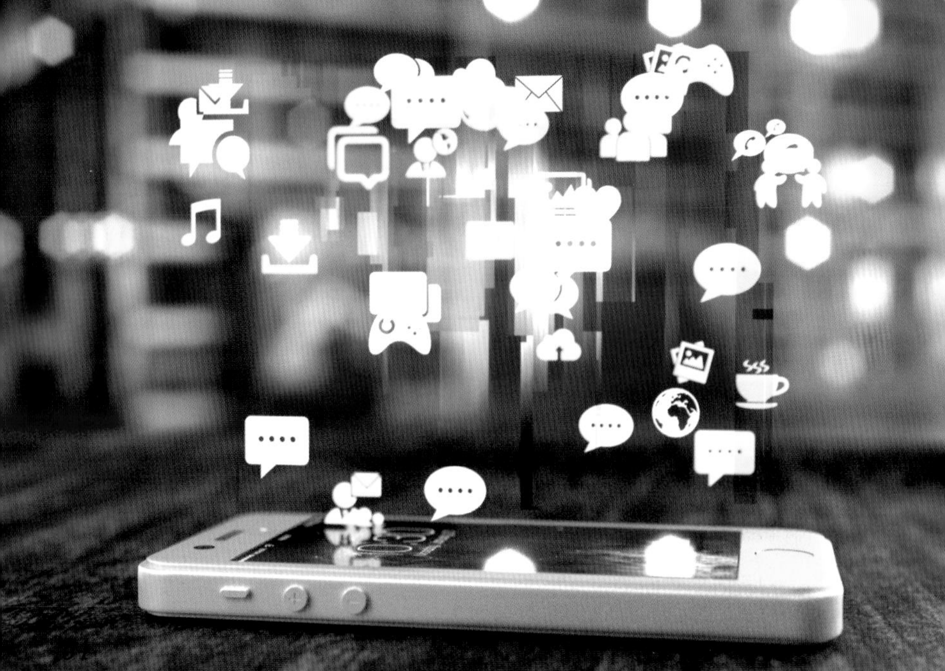

4) Compensation Plan Knowledge & Product Knowledge

Without looking, do you know what it takes to get to the next title? The more you know about each advancement and what it takes to get there, the better you'll be able to make important decisions that actually get you there.

This goes hand-in-hand with Strategic Building. The more you know about the Compensation Plan, the more you can assess ***where*** and ***what*** you need to advance your rank. By becoming a Comp Plan genius, you'll soon be able to see areas of your organization that are weak or that could use some sprucing.

5) Strategic Building

Do you know the benefits of Stacking, Duplicating, and Strategic Building? Thought so. Your Young Living journey will often start with you not knowing what you don't know. That's okay. But, it really helps you to connect with those who do understand the Compensation Plan in great detail. If you're at all cloudy on the subject, you'll want to find a business buddy who knows it. They can be part of a Facebook group, someone on your immediate team, someone in your upline, or someone who simply would be willing to help you get clear in no uncertain terms.

Where to begin? Change your ***flat*** thinking to ***stack*** thinking. Think in terms of depth. The magic number of first-level distributors on your team is 6. Once you have this basic number, it can take you all the way to Royal Crown Diamond. But, you don't want just anyone filling up those six spots.

Here's how it works. You may approach a less-than-fully-motivated business leader and ask them if they would consider allowing you to bring a motivated person on underneath them. This helps you fill out the team. Sometimes, a member might not initially take to the business-building motivators that motivate others. If you think there's still potential, you can place someone motivated underneath them so that they have a running partner in the business. They each can gain from helping the other out. It may be just what the under-motivated person needs to get things into gear. It might be the gentle push or the motivator to draw out leadership in this person. It may create a healthy competition, but you have to do this with care and knowledge of personalities and how they fit together.

Strategic building is also about creating the right touch-point contact, communication and encouragement. Every person on your team is unique. Each member will be motivated just a little differently. Recognize this quickly and support that person by giving them personalized encouragement, positivity, and acknowledgement. Strategic building isn't about moving pawns on a board. It's about knowing and understanding people—quickly getting familiar with their talents and natural abilities—and using that information to make the whole team more successful as a whole. Everyone adds value. Figure out the best way to leverage that value to ensure your whole organization grows and moves forward.

Keep in mind that some of the best leaders will sometimes place their own new members under your level one. If they make that request, try to accommodate it. It may be a great thing to help you. They're looking out for the team as a whole. Rather than harboring any resentment, ask them to explain how to do the same type of stacking for the team you are trying to build. Let them know that you are perfectly willing to take direction and learn. Ultimately, it is your business, your setup, and your final decision.

Lastly, the best builders know that Essential Rewards works better than anything else for motivating consistent PV. Who doesn't want to be rewarded with their favorite lifestyle products? This creates a strong circle in your team: they use the products, like the products, share the products, and earn more of their favorites.

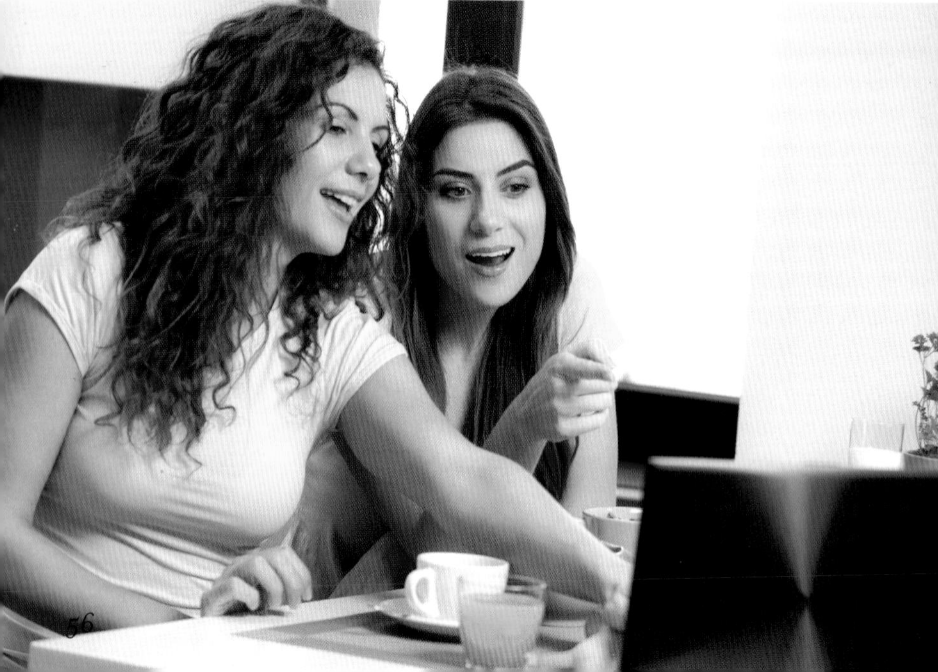

Questions to consider as you determine your own stacking structure:

Who is in your Level One?

Who is in your Level Two?

Who is your number one go-getter?

Who seems to know everybody?

Who seems to be able to get to know anybody?

Who has a contact list that seems never-ending?

Who is a wait-and-see type of personality? (Remember: if often takes 3-8 weeks for an analytical person to decide what to do.)

Who are the people you can help?

Who are the people who can help you?

Who is best at recruiting/customer setting?

Who is best at recruiting/customer closing?

Who is best at training?

Who is best at celebrating and recognizing?

Who is interested in ordering every month?

Who is interested in getting their products for free?

Who is interested in building a business?

LEARN MORE...

This is just the tip of the iceberg when it comes to all of the possibilities for using essential oils. And, these oils are only a fraction of the collection. Talk to your local Young Living member about all of the collection as well as discounts and rewards for using Young Living products.

SHARE MORE...

Life Science Publishing and Products has everything you need to explore the history, the traditions, the research, the science, and the uses for all essential oils. Visit www.discoverlsp.com to learn how you can make the most of every essential oil single or blend. Whether you need books or tools for your home, glassware for your business, or brochures for helping you share, consider Life Science Publishing & Products your perfect partner.

Content herein derives from the Essential Oil Desk Reference, also owned and published by Life Science Publishing.

Life Science Publishing is the publisher of this handbook. Life Science Publishing is not responsible for its content. The information contained herein is for educational purposes only. It is not provided to diagnose, prescribe, or treat any condition of the body. The information in this handbook should not be used as a substitute for medical counseling with a health professional. Neither the author nor the publisher accepts responsibility for such use.